Men's Health

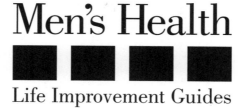

Life Improvement Guides

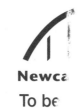
Food Smart

A Man's Plan
to Fuel Up for
Peak Performance

by Jeff Bredenberg, Alisa Bauman
and the Editors of **Men'sHealth** Books

Rodale Press, Inc.
Emmaus, Pennsylvania

Notice

This book is intended as a reference volume only, not as a medical manual. The information given here is designed to help you make informed decisions about your health. It is not intended as a substitute for any treatment that may have been prescribed by your doctor. If you suspect that you have a medical problem, we urge you to seek competent medical help.

Library of Congress Cataloging-in-Publication Data

Bredenberg, Jeff.
Food smart: a man's plan to fuel up for peak performance / by Jeff Bredenberg, Alisa Bauman and the editors of
    Men's Health Books.
        p.   cm.—(Men's health life improvement guides)
    Includes index.
    ISBN 0-87596-280-7 paperback
    1.   Men—Nutrition. I. Bauman, Alisa. II. Men's Health Books. III. Title. IV. Series.
RA777.8.B74 1996
613.2'081—dc20   96–816

Distributed in the book trade by St. Martin's Press

2 4 6 8 10 9 7 5 3 1   paperback

— OUR MISSION —

We publish books that empower people's lives.

RODALE BOOKS

Food Smart Editorial Staff

Senior Managing Editor: **Neil Wertheimer**

Senior Editor: **Jack Croft**

Writers: **Jeff Bredenberg, Alisa Bauman, Jack Croft, Stephen C. George**

Associate Art Director: **Faith Hague**

Book and Cover Designer: **John Herr**

Cover Photographer: **Walter Smith**

Photo Editor: **Susan Pollack**

Illustrators: **Thomas P. Aczel, J. Andrew Brubaker, Mark Matcho, David Q. Pryor**

Studio Manager: **Joe Golden**

Technical Artist: **David Q. Pryor**

Layout Artist: **Mary Brundage**

Assistant Research Manager: **Carol Svec**

Researchers and Fact-Checkers: **Christine Dreisbach, Jan Eickmeier, Karen Marmarus, Deborah Pedron, Sally A. Reith, Bernadette Sukley, Margo Trott, John Waldron**

Copy Editors: **Amy K. Fisher, John D. Reeser**

Production Manager: **Helen Clogston**

Manufacturing Coordinator: **Melinda B. Rizzo**

Office Staff: **Roberta Mulliner, Julie Kehs, Bernadette Sauerwine, Mary Lou Stephen**

Rodale Health and Fitness Books

Vice-President and Editorial Director: **Debora T. Yost**

Art Director: **Jane Colby Knutila**

Research Manager: **Ann Gossy Yermish**

Copy Manager: **Lisa D. Andruscavage**

Contents

Introduction

Fear No Food

It's never been easier to eat healthy. It's also never been harder.

We have more choices than our grandparents ever could have imagined. Thanks to innovations in technology and transportation, fresh fruit and vegetables abound year-round. Red meat has grown decidedly leaner, and it's amazing what you can do with turkey or chicken these days. New low-fat but delicious versions of our old lard-laden favorites hit the supermarket shelves almost every day. And even fast-food joints and convenience stores have started offering items that won't clog your arteries before you hit the door.

The problem is that many of us continue to literally live off the fat of the land. Nutritional ignorance is indeed bliss. But it can also be deadly. We now know beyond any reasonable doubt that eating a diet high in fruits, vegetables and carbohydrates such as pasta and rice provides protection against the diseases that kill men most frequently. Cancer. Heart attack. Diabetes.

Living longer is one thing. But if it means taking a vow of perpetual blandness—"I swear, never again will any food with taste pass these lips"—most guys aren't sure it's worth it.

Neither are we. Fortunately, that's not our choice. Nutritional knowledge is power—power to make choices that enable us to eat for pure pleasure *and* good health. The book you're now holding in your hands will give you that power.

First, a few brief words about what this book isn't. It's not a cookbook. If you're looking for recipes, you'll have to look elsewhere. (Although if you stick with us to the "Buying Cookbooks" chapter in Part One, you'll find some great recommendations. And we do tell you how to make a delectable dish with mealworms in the "Condiments" chapter in Part Two.) It's also not a sermon. We're not going to harangue you to turn to a life of sacrifice and self-denial. We're not about to live like that, and neither should you. Perhaps most importantly, it's not a diet book. Diets don't work. Period. If you're looking for a quick fix, you're in the wrong place.

Food Smart is more than just the title of this volume in the *Men's Health* Life Improvement Guides series. It will be the phrase others use to describe you after you've finished reading it.

As with the other books in the series, you'll find each page chock-full of down-to-earth, no-nonsense, let's-do-it-now health information researched and written exclusively for men. This book goes where men go. To the bar. To the ballpark. To the movies. It offers smart strategies for different cuisines while clueing you in on how to get the best meals at your favorite fast-food restaurants and convenience stores. It will go with you on the plane and in your car, and offers valuable tips on how to eat for specific goals ranging from improving your sex life to boosting your brainpower.

Food is meant to be savored, not shoveled. Eating doesn't merely fulfill a biological need. It should be a sensual experience, a lifelong adventure. Our motto is "Fear No Food," and on the pages that follow we hope to open your taste buds to the truly incredible array of surprises food has to offer.

Bon appétit.

Neil Wertheimer
Senior Managing Editor, *Men's Health* Books

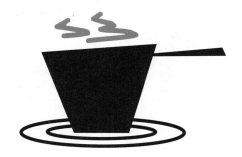

Part One

What a Man Needs

How We Eat

Too Much, and Not Enough

How does it feel to be wealthy?

Okay, maybe you're more a Rocky than a Rockefeller. But it's likely that to some degree you're wallowing in America's astounding economic success over the last century.

Compared to the rest of the world, our food is cheaper—particularly meats, restaurant meals and processed foods. At dinner we can afford to give meat and cheese star billing as opposed to, say, the rice commonly found on Asian tables. We've made dessert an indelible finale to the appetizer-salad-entrée progression. Shoot, even the famed pastry chefs of Europe are only trotted out for special occasions. Day in and day out, those poor mopes overseas suffer with only fruit to top off their meals.

Americans also revel in labor-saving machinery, such as power tools, vacuum cleaners, salad spinners and riding lawn mowers. Driving a car is cheap in the United States, and our cities are designed to accommodate swarms of autos—unlike the claustrophobic lanes of Old World cultures that are more suited to foot traffic and bicycles.

But before you pat yourself on the back, pat yourself on the belly. Whatcha got there? A tractor-tread array of rippling abs? Or a balloon tire?

Chances are, it's the latter. Three-quarters of American men age 25 and over are above their recommended weight range, according to the Prevention Index, which tracks healthful behavior in the population. And being overweight is a complicating factor in a number of the nation's top killer diseases, like cancer, heart dis-

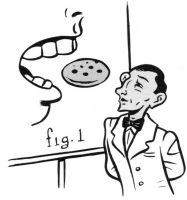

fig. 1

ease and stroke. In fact, those three diseases account for 75 percent of the deaths in the United States each year. And each of those maladies, scientists say, is directly related to how you eat.

In that light, our steak-and-leisure legacy seems more like a curse.

The Balancing Act

While most Americans actually do know a thing or two about nutrition, a study by CDB Research and Consulting in New York City found that 69 percent of men say they find it very hard to eat a balanced diet. Two thirds of Americans—more of them men than women—say they're confused by news reports about what foods to avoid. You know:

- "Fat Packs a Punch in Kung Pao Chicken." *But I thought Chinese food was healthy!*
- "Just Say Ciao to Fettuccine Alfredo." *But isn't pasta good for you?*

What's launching some of our favorite foods into the screamer headlines? For the most part: fat.

Red meat is the biggest source of saturated fat in an American man's diet. That's the stuff that stops up your arteries. What's more, eating a diet heavy in red meat and light on vegetables and fruits puts you at greater risk of getting colon and prostate cancer—which, after lung cancer, are the two cancers that kill the most men. If you have red meat five times a week, you're four times more likely to get colon cancer than if you eat it just once a month.

The Food and Drug Administration's Daily Values recommend that you get no more than 30 percent of your calories from fat. (Some experts suggest that 20 percent or less would be better.) The Daily Values are calculated on 10 percent of your calories coming from protein and 60 percent from carbohydrates.

On the average, we fall on the dangerous side of those recommendations. Men between the ages of 20 and 60 get about 34 percent of their calories from fat, 47 percent from carbohydrates, around 15 percent from protein and 4 percent from alcohol. (A note about alcohol: People tend to fudge when survey staffers ask them how much they drink. Four percent of calories for the average guy in his thirties would be more than half an ounce of alcohol. That's a bit more than you would get in a standard 12-ounce beer.)

Grasping the dietary numbers is no picnic, but for many men the hardest part of eating well is overcoming deeply ingrained attitudes about food. "People hold up ideals, which are socially and culturally set standards of what is a good meal," says Jeffery Sobal, Ph.D., a medical sociologist who specializes in nutrition research at Cornell University in Ithaca, New York. "These are root orientations that people use in deciding what to eat—and how to rationalize why they didn't choose something else."

Another confounding part of the equation: Men don't have a good handle on *how much* they're eating of certain foods. A survey commissioned by the Livestock and Meat Board showed that most guys believe their eating closely follows the recommendations of the government's Food Guide Pyramid. While men, on average, think they're getting 2.3 servings a day of dairy foods, they actually get 1.2. (Two to three servings are recommended.) And while they think they're getting 2.1 servings of fruit per day, they're actually getting only 1. (Two to four servings are best.) Now let's give credit where credit's due: Men think they're getting 2.4 servings of vegetables a day, and that's accurate (although 3 to 5 servings are recommended).

A Matter of Taste

Why do we decide to eat the foods that we do? The reasons are complex indeed. Among the influences:

- **Personal preference: Maybe you just love garlicky Indian food.**
- **Tradition: Lasagna's been on the family table since Grandpa came over on the boat.**
- **Social interaction: Let's invite Sam over, order a pizza and turn on the football game.**
- **Convenience: Half a bagel, a quick slurp of coffee and you're out the door in the morning.**
- **Habit: What? I *always* eat peanut butter and jelly for lunch.**
- **Belief: I'm giving up meat for Lent.**

What's missing? Oh, yeah! Nutrition. Certain foods will keep me healthy.

All of the above reasons are understandable influences on what you eat, but nutrition needs to play a major role no matter what your mood or situation.

A note about those ranges of servings: When health officials say adults should eat 5 to 9 servings of fruits and vegetables, they intend for men to gravitate toward the higher end because they eat more food than women. So their total of 3 or 4 servings a day of fruits and vegetables falls far short of the ideal of 9.

Enough of the finger-wagging. There are also bright spots in the report. A survey by the Calorie Control Council shows these trends.

- Seventy-four percent of American men say they're eating a more healthful diet than they were three years ago.
- Fifty-seven percent of men say they always try to check nutrition labels for fat content.
- And 52 percent of men say they always try to check the nutrition label for calorie content.

How We Should Eat

Struggling with Food? Get a Lifestyle

Did you play jackstraws as a kid? You take a handful of thin sticks and let them fall into a heap. Then you try to lift one stick at a time without moving any of the others. It's tough: You'd think they were all inter-connected, the way they teeter and turn and slide at the slightest touch.

Nutrition is a lot like that. When you read about the best ways to feed yourself, the same advice keeps popping up in a number of different contexts. Want to protect yourself from colon cancer? Get plenty of fiber from fruits, vegetables, legumes and grains. Want to lower your cholesterol? Fiber again. Want to control your weight? Those high-fiber foods you're packing away move more slowly through the digestive tract, making you feel less hungry. Meanwhile, foods that give you lots of fiber also give you less of the stuff you want to avoid, like fat, cholesterol, refined sugar and salt.

The key approaches to healthy and happy eating are not so much brilliant, independent ideas as they are pieces of the same puzzle, end-lessly interlocking. If it sounds like feeding yourself well is an overwhelming task, relax. We're not necessarily talking about radical lifestyle changes. Scien-tists say even modest adjust-ments in diet will substantially reduce your risk of developing some of the nation's most com-mon men killers. (Although the focus of this book is food, the same goes for taking up exercise.)

"We have a serious problem in this country. One out of every three Americans is overweight, and that represents a big increase in just the last decade," says Jayne Hurley, senior nutritionist at the Center for Science in the Public Interest in Washington, D.C., and a writer for the *Nutrition Action Healthletter.* "We have heart disease, cancer and a number of other diet-related diseases as our big killers. In fact, as many people die each year from a lack of exercise and bad diet—a combination of those two—as from cigarette smoking."

Here's a rundown of central themes that will pop up repeatedly in the coming chapters of this book. As you read on, you'll learn why these approaches work and how to make them a pleasurable part of your life.

Trim the fat. Fat in the diet contributes to heart disease, cancer, diabetes and obesity. Saturated fat, the kind found primarily in animal foods, is the most harmful kind. So limit your intake of red meat, whole milk, cheese and other fatty foods.

Build on the pyramid. This is one pyramid scheme you can take to the bank. The U.S. government's Food Guide Pyramid recom-mends a diet heavy in grains, fruits and vegeta-bles, moderate consumption of meat and dairy products and limited use of sweets, fats and oils.

Tune up with carbs. The complex car-bohydrates you get from grains, fruits and veg-etables are a top-notch, low-fat energy source.

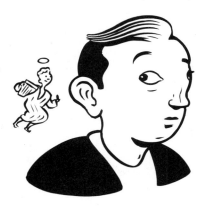

Favor fiber. High-fiber plant foods, like whole-grain bread, bran cereal and beans, improve digestion, lower blood cholesterol and lower your risk of cancer and heart disease.

Branch out. There's safety in numbers—that is, eating a great number of different foods. For one thing, each food has its strong points.

Eating a wide variety of foods gives you a broad, protective mosaic of nutrients. Besides, life gets more interesting when you eat something new occasionally. So fear no food.

Take out insurance. It's best to get your vitamins and minerals from the foods you eat, nutrition experts say. One reason: Scientists suspect foods contain protective substances—phytochemicals and others we haven't even identified yet. But, okay, this is the real world. If your dietary program bears the inscription "Coming Soon: Massive Improvements," you might want to take a vitamin and mineral supplement for insurance until you can find the produce section of your grocery store. Just remember, supplements are not a more-is-better thing. Some vitamins are toxic in high doses.

Set limits. Limit your consumption of refined sugar, salt and alcohol. Refined sugar, the stuff you get in candy and packaged snacks, gives you "empty" calories—no beneficial nutrition—and plays hell with your metabolism. Excessive salt intake can contribute to high blood pressure. High alcohol intake increases the risk of cancer and interferes with nutrient absorption.

Control your weight.
Seriously overweight people are more likely to get heart attacks, stroke and diabetes. Weight loss is by no means a simple issue. But basically, your body weight will hold stable if the energy you consume from food equals the energy you expend in your daily activities. If you take in more calories than you burn, you gain weight. If you burn more calories than you take in, you lose weight.

Deep-six dieting. Diets don't work. You choose foods from a skimpy list, wrestle with deprivation and maybe slurp some milky

Conquering Food Fears

Afraid to try new foods?

Researchers have studied the problem and they have suggestions. U.S. Army and Finnish researchers selected 121 people to participate in a study. Sixty of them were "neophilics," meaning they love to try new things. Sixty-one were "neophobics," meaning they don't like new things at all. The test subjects were introduced to four foods in unmarked containers, two that were unfamiliar and two that would prove familiar: a Finnish pudding, a Finnish nonalcoholic beer, apple butter and root beer. The hitch: A third of the people were given no information about the food, another group was given only product names for the four foods and the others were told in detail about the foods' ingredients and their uses.

The test subjects, fearful and fearless alike, liked the foods more when they had information about them. The neophobics hit a "ceiling," however, and never totally warmed up to the novel Finnish foods.

So to help yourself overcome an initial dislike to a new food, the researchers concluded:

- **Get all the information you can about the food.**
- **Increase your exposure to it—look at it, smell it and taste it.**
- **Draw parallels between the new food and foods you're comfortable with—between the Finnish pudding and apple butter, for instance.**

substance sold to you as part of a miracle weight-loss plan. Your weight drops. You return to your old eating pattern and soon you're back in the closet looking for your "big" pants.

Healthy weight loss is done gradually, as part of a lifestyle change. Eat when you're hungry, but eat low-fat, high-carbohydrate foods. And exercise.

The Truth about Calorie Counting

Hint: You Won't Need Your Calculator

If you've ever tried a low-calorie diet, maybe you can sympathize with the fellows in the Minnesota Experiment.

Near the end of World War II, 32 conscientious objectors spent six months on a semistarvation diet. They hoped to shed light on the problem of world hunger and provide the knowledge necessary to rehabilitate malnourished concentration camp victims. The volunteers consumed an average of 1,570 calories a day, less than half their consumption during the preceding three-month "control" period. The men were required by University of Minnesota researchers to lose an average of 24 percent of their body weight.

They started out as an educated, jovial and idealistic bunch. After six months of self-induced famine, they were a hyperirritable, nail-biting, back-biting, plate-licking bunch of obsessives who had lost all interest in their original altruism. They lost 30 percent of their strength, their metabolisms dropped 40 percent and they performed their work assignments poorly. The volunteers spent three more months easing toward unrestricted eating again but then found themselves gobbling 5,200 calories a day and as many as three lunches back-to-back.

War may be hell, but severe dieting is no picnic either. By trying to subsist on something like carrot sticks and lettuce, you're actually sabotaging your own efforts to trim fat from your waistline, scientists say. You're entering a morass of frustration, guilt, berserk appetites and binges. Then, feeling weak and deprived, you're likely to revert with a vengeance to your old eating style, gaining more weight than ever.

"Some research suggests that restrained eating may be unhealthful in itself," says Cornell University's Dr. Jeffery Sobal. "If you try to live a restrained life, you are eventually going to fail and you are going to get fatter."

The Real Battle of the Bulge

When you diet, you aren't just combating a few pounds of fat. You're squaring off against a large, sophisticated organism that doesn't take kindly to starvation. On-again-off-again dieting trains your enzymes to take a defensive posture: They start socking away fat whenever the body threatens to lose weight, says Michael Colgan, Ph.D., president of the Colgan Institute of Nutritional Science in San Diego and author of *Optimum Sports Nutrition.*

"I think a classic example is the 'boomerang' dieter," says Dr. Colgan. "He's terribly overweight and he can't eat a thing. If he eats a peanut, he tends to gain weight, because the body won't let him use it for energy. He has all of this active enzyme, lipoprotein lipase, rushing about grabbing fat molecules. And there's another enzyme in the liver that's continually trying to turn carbohydrates into fat as well. People force themselves into this diet corner all of the time, and I think the diet industry has been responsible for teaching Americans to do this."

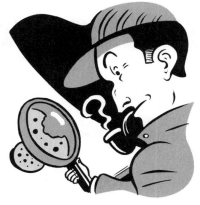

Does this mean calorie-counting is dead? In terms of crash dieting, yes. But you still need to understand what calories are and where you're getting them.

Pump Up the Volume

What in the world is a calorie anyway? Calories (what scientists formally call kilocalories) are a measure of heat energy provided by food. The 100 calories in two tablespoons of sugar, for example, is enough to turn 4 cups of ice into boiling water. The calories in one tablespoon of fat would do the same. So would the calories in 4½ cups of shredded cabbage.

That difference in volume is crucial. It's why nutrition experts say you can control your weight by gravitating toward whole grains, fruits and vegetables. You can pretty much eat all you want of those foods without accumulating excess calories that will be converted to fat. A one-ounce snippet of pork chop will give you a quick 100 calories, and you'd undoubtedly eat more than that in one sitting. But imagine eating 100 calories' worth of asparagus: You'd have to wolf down 25 spears, an unlikely feat.

Aside from the wonderful nutrients you get from grains, fruits and vegetables, you also need their bulk just to alert you when it's time to stop eating. Experiments have demonstrated that when people are allowed to eat until they feel full, the fellows who go for high-fat foods rack up more calories per meal than those who eat low-fat, even if the meals are equally tasty. This means that you do not have a built-in calorie meter that tells you when to stop scarfing ribs or doughnuts. Fullness, from the bulk of the food you have eaten, persuades you to put the fork down.

You can measure your success by belt notches. Each pound of fat you gain or lose represents 3,500 calories. This means that consuming just 100 excess calories a day will layer 11 pounds of fat on your frame in the course of a year.

Losing weight, of course, works in the reverse: When you regularly use more energy than you take in, the pounds melt away. But remember that the best weight-reduction plans are gradual, involving sensible eating and exercise.

So quit depriving yourself. Stop trying to count every calorie. Heap your plate with low-fat, high-carbohydrate, high-fiber foods, like potatoes, whole-grain breads and pastas, beans and lentils, apples, bananas, melons and skim-milk products. And once you're eating healthier fare, see if you can handle this one simple rule: When you feel full, stop eating.

Running on Empty

If you think "sugar-free" means you don't have to pay for the sweet stuff in your soda, you're likely to get mighty confused by the term "empty calories."

Sorry, but it doesn't mean those calories don't count. In fact, it means just the opposite, says Liz Applegate, Ph.D., nutrition editor for *Runner's World* magazine. Cola is considered an empty-calorie drink because it offers little else of value beyond calories. Unlike an apple, for instance, cola doesn't contain vitamins, minerals or fiber, Dr. Applegate notes.

And to make matters worse, those empty calories crowd out foods that do provide nutrients. Once you fill up on potato chips and soda, there's no room left for the good stuff, Dr. Applegate warns.

Her advice: Eat empty-calorie foods in moderation and be food smart. Look for nutrient-dense foods—fruits, vegetables, low- or nonfat dairy products and whole grains—that give your body far more than just more calories.

Different Folks, Different Forks

Hey, Guy, You're One-of-a-Kind

Which of the following are members of your species: Arnold Schwarzenegger or Spike Lee? Jimmy Smits or Lyle Lovett?

The answer, of course, is "all of the above."

The world is crawling with some six billion Homo sapiens, and no two of us are identical chemically, psychologically, in preferences, in talent, in political beliefs or in shape. That's why there are so many kinds of mouthwash, athletic shoes and tax forms.

And that's why there are so many different ways of eating. Your tastes, and your body's needs, are one-of-a-kind.

The difference in body chemistry is no trifling matter. The concept of "biochemical individuality" was pioneered more than 40 years ago by University of Texas scientist Roger Williams, considered to be the father of modern nutrition science. It has been demonstrated, for instance, that some animals need 20 times more vitamin C than others. Today, scientists know that human needs for vitamins, minerals and other nutrients vary greatly.

"Williams started looking at different enzyme levels. He saw that they're all totally different," says Michael J. González, D.Sc., Ph.D., assistant professor of nutritional biochemistry and advanced nutrition at the University of Puerto Rico Medical Sciences Campus School of Public Health in San Juan. "People can be functional but have different levels of efficiency in their enzymes. It's true

for medicines, too—a medicine could help one person and be toxic to another person. And in nutrition what helps one person with a problem might not necessarily help another one."

One glance around the locker room tells you there's no standard-issue body. America may have a fixation on body weight, but the degree to which you tip the scales is not giving you a complete reading on your health status.

Oh, a common height-and-weight table will tell you that if you're 35 or older and stand 5 feet 11 inches tall, your ideal weight is 151 to 194 pounds. A guy with dense bones and muscles like Apollo could be "overweight" by that measure. On the other hand, a Bacchus-belly couch potato with little muscle and loads of fat might fall smack in the middle of that ideal-weight range. Need we say which guy is healthier?

The issue that's more important than weight, then, is how much fat is hanging from your skeleton—and where it's located. Men tend to collect fat around the abdomen, and that's the most dangerous kind. A beer belly greatly increases your risk of heart disease, stroke, diabetes and high blood pressure.

The Role of Genetics

Scientists say genetics can influence how susceptible or resistant you are to gaining body fat. Studies show that identical twins (with the same genetic makeup) are twice as likely to have the same weight as fraternal twins (who are less genetically similar). This applies even when the twins are raised apart.

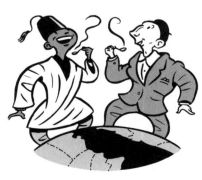

Genetics may also influence your metabolic rate and your body's inclination to store fat, which are factors in weight gain.

So, yes, you're dealt some cards you have no control over.

But that's just a starting point, not the end-all. It's up to you to assess your body's needs and fashion a nutrition program that fits.

"Your body chemistry is affected by your choices," says Dr. Michael Colgan of the Colgan Institute of Nutritional Science. "Take the example of a man who is overweight because of poor diet and insufficient exercise. This individual carries these few extra pounds in large part because he likes to have dessert or he likes his beer. His overweight condition is not a genetic problem. Contrary to commonly held beliefs, only about 1 percent or less of the population are genetically overweight."

Flagging Bad Habits

No matter what your ethnic heritage, any of the common eating patterns across the world can be adapted to high-energy, heart-healthy, cancer-battling nutrition. The general strategy: Keep fat consumption down by limiting such foods as butter, margarine, mayonnaise, fatty meats and whole milk. Here are just a few examples.

If your main ethnic influence is northern European, you may think a dream dinner includes a large slab of roast meat, side dishes of mashed potatoes and boiled cabbage, bread and fruit pie for dessert. Well, that gives you a good supply of protein and other nutrients that come with meat, but unfortunately, it's a high-fat diet that's low in the fiber, vitamins and minerals that come with fruits and vegetables. So take a smaller portion of meat and eat more whole grains, fruits and vegetables.

If you're fond of Jewish cuisine, reduce the chicken fat used in cooking and fry potato pancakes on nonstick pans instead of in oil.

It Takes Two

If you have trouble choking down your broccoli, blame Mom and Dad. Okay, you may be a wimp, too, but we're giving you the benefit of the doubt. That's because nutrition researchers are discovering that the distaste for certain flavor compounds in foods can be inherited.

Researchers at the University of Cincinnati tested 14 pairs of identical twins and 21 pairs of same-sex fraternal twins for their taste preferences. They ranged in age from 9 to 18 years and each pair was reared in the same home, so the environmental influences were the same. Identical twins have the same genetic makeup, while fraternal twins do not. Therefore, when the identical twins showed an above-average pattern of agreement about the taste of a food, that indicated an inherited trait.

Tests showed a genetic factor in their preference for broccoli, chicken, cottage cheese, orange juice, sweetened cereal and hamburger.

Even the genetically less similar fraternal twins in the Cincinnati test showed substantial agreement on a preference for one food. Big surprise: snack cake.

Keep the bagels and lox, but skip the cream cheese.

A real Mexican meal is typically a bean stew, meat, rice, tortillas and salsa—not bad at all. It's the Mexican restaurants in the United States that lard the cuisine down with such items as fried tortillas, cheese, sour cream and guacamole. So go back to the roots, amigo, and give priority to the beans, rice, lettuce and soft corn or flour tortillas.

The bottom line: The U.S. government's Food Guide Pyramid—emphasizing lots of grains, fruits and vegetables and limited use of fat and sweets—is an eating strategy that can be adapted to any culture.

Key Nutrients for Men

Better Living through Chemistry

As the manager of a complex organization, would you hire staffers who all had identical skills? No, there are too many diverse jobs to be done, ranging from reception to accounting to production. Would you hire randomly? Of course not. You'd carefully match skills to the work that needs doing.

So here you are, the CEO of a human body, and your body has some needs.

- Energy
- Building materials
- Chemicals to regulate vital processes

You have to meet those needs with the stuff you stick in your mouth. To succeed, you'll require lots of different foods and a wise selection process. Which means you need to know the "résumé"—the beneficial content—of a food before you pass it between your teeth.

The chemicals in food that help us live and grow are called nutrients. The essential nutrients are the ones your body can't make on its own or can't make enough of, and you'd die without them: carbohydrates, protein, vitamins, minerals, water and fat. (We've honored fat with a chapter of its own.) Fiber is another crucial, yet sorely neglected, factor in the diet, so we'll take a look at that, too.

Understanding nutrients does not require an advanced degree in chemistry. You won't have to tape a cheat sheet to your wrist before you cruise the supermarket. But you do want a basic understanding of where to get your nutrients and what amounts you need.

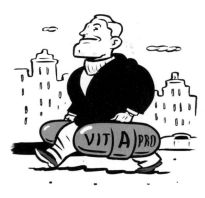

The more you learn about the sources and importance of these nutrients, the more clearly you'll understand why nutrition experts are so enthusiastic about fruits, vegetables and whole grains. And the more you'll understand how processing weakens food by whittling away nutrients.

"I think we have what *Time* magazine referred to as a green wave of people who are buying almost exclusively organic foods. These consumers are looking to whole grains and vegetables as the basis of their diet," says Dr. Michael Colgan of the Colgan Institute of Nutritional Science. "And I think by the year 2000, if we keep putting out the right sort of information, we'll have a much healthier nation."

Carbohydrates: Power to the People

Sure, you can burn a number of substances for energy—fat, protein, and even alcohol. But your body doesn't suffer these fuels gladly. Scarfing a lot of fat can lead to nasty diseases, like cancer and heart disease. When your body has to rely on protein for energy, it's not satisfied with the meat and eggs you eat—it starts dismantling your muscle tissue, too. And alcohol is a nutritional bully: Not only does it feed you "empty" calories, meaning you get zip for sustenance, but it also plays hell with your liver, your brain and the nutritional metabolism in every shred of tissue.

So it's no wonder that you hear so much glowing praise for carbohydrates. They're a top-notch energy source, and the foods that tend to provide them—fruits, vegetables, beans and grains—are low in fat and high in fiber.

"There is a strong drive toward reducing fat intake, and

the only way to do that and to maintain an adequate amount of caloric intake is to increase the consumption of carbohydrates," says Benjamin Caballero, M.D., Ph.D., director of the Center for Human Nutrition at Johns Hopkins University in Baltimore. "So carbohydrates are becoming more and more important precisely because we need to check the amount of fat we eat every day."

Any plant you'd care to eat has carbohydrate in it. Remember seventh-grade science? During photosynthesis, plants combine carbon with a molecule of water. Get it? A *carbon* that's been *hydrated*. This has been our primary energy source since our ancestors peeled their first banana. Oh, during the 1950s many people mistakenly thought high-carb foods were fattening, but by the mid-1970s mainstream scientists were saying that a diet high in complex carbohydrates could prevent a number of chronic diseases.

Develop a Complex

Before you reflexively reach for the channel changer to zap to another chapter, rest assured that there's really nothing all that complex about complex carbohydrates. In fact, carbohydrates are divided into two straightforward categories.

• Simple carbohydrates. These are small molecules that are rapidly absorbed. The most common is table sugar (sucrose). The most common natural simple carbohydrate is fructose, also present in most soft drinks, says Dr. Caballero. Most of us, unfortunately, vacuum down far too much refined sugar, in the form of candy and other sweets.

• Complex carbohydrates. These are also called starches, which come in vegetables,

Processing Goes against the Grain

Fans of Howdy Doody and Buffalo Bob knew how to build strong bodies 12 different ways: Eat white bread. Bread comes from flour, flour comes from grain, and we modern guys want those carbohydrates from grain, right? White bread even comes enriched with nutrients. So what's the problem?

The milling process. Any way you slice it, even enriched, processed bread is no competition for unrefined, whole-grain bread. Processing strips the bran and germ from the grain, meaning a host of important nutrients are lost. Manufacturers typically toss back in iron, thiamin, riboflavin and niacin, but a lot of good stuff is still left on the cutting room floor, including fiber, magnesium, zinc and vitamin B_6.

"White flour is processed death—the body looks at it as if it was sugar," says Dr. Michael Colgan. "So-called 'enriched flour' is exactly the same. In many enriched flours, manufacturers take out something like 40 different vitamin and mineral substances and put back in 8 at the most."

At the Colgan Institute of Nutritional Science, Dr. Colgan found healthy weevils that had invaded some whole-grain flour. He put them into a large plastic bag along with a couple of processed Italian loaves and supplied them with a steady trickle of air.

"The weevils died," he says. "If weevils can't live on it, you can't live on it, either."

fruits, beans, pastas, breads and other grain foods. Starches are huge molecules made up of simple sugars. It takes your body longer to break them down, which moderates the flow of blood sugar into your bloodstream.

"It makes a big difference. Not every carbohydrate is the same to your body," says Dr. Caballero. "When you eat something, there's a big increase in your blood sugar. The height of that peak is now considered a very important factor in diabetes and other problems, so we want to have a food that has the same amount of energy but does not create such a high peak of blood sugar."

Because the sugar from complex carbohydrates reaches the bloodstream more gradually, it does not require a large surge in insulin, the hormone that removes blood sugar from the blood and socks it away in various cells. "So those are the ones we need to aim for in our diet: whole-wheat bread, oatmeal, pastas—anything that has starch in it," says Dr. Caballero.

The typical male between ages 20 and 50 gets about 47 percent of his calories from carbohydrates. Americans were getting 56 percent in the early 1900s. The proportion of complex carbohydrates in the American diet, however, has plunged by more than 30 percent since the turn of the century, while consumption of sugars has soared. Nutrition experts recommend that 55 to 60 percent of total calories come from carbohydrates, and that no more than 10 percent be from added sugar.

Some research is challenging the idea that simple sugars hit your bloodstream more quickly than starches. But even if it's proven that simple and complex carbohydrates are metabolized similarly, the advice about consuming them isn't likely to change. The complex carbs will still be praised for the beneficial nutrients that accompany them, and simple carbs will still be infamous for bringing empty calories and extra fat to the table.

The Athletic Edge

Carbohydrates may be the second-most-talked-about thing in the locker room. Open any nutrition book written in the last few years and you're likely to find a strategy for athletes called carbohydrate loading.

While there are lots of theories swirling around carbo loading, it basically involves feasting on complex carbohydrates, like spaghetti and bread, for a few days before a big endurance feat. This helps you store extra glycogen in your muscles—a reserve tank of fuel.

A high-carb diet is often associated with steady, long-haul events, like marathon running, but scientists are discovering it also provides an edge in sports such as soccer that require extreme, intermittent bursts of energy.

At the University of Queensland in Brisbane, Australia, for instance, researchers fed 14 young men just a moderate amount of carbohydrates for three days. Then the men exercised on stationary cycles in five all-out, one-minute bursts with five minutes rest between each session. Researchers then divided the men into three groups and fed them for three more days on diets either high in carbohydrates (83 percent of their energy), moderate (58 percent) or low (12 percent). When they were retested, those on the high-carb diet did 5.6 percent more work during the all-out exercise. The moderate group did 2.3 percent more work, and the low group did 5.4 percent less work.

While carbohydrates clearly provide an athletic edge, all-out, scientifically done carbo loading is only a benefit to highly trained athletes who work their gas gauges down to zero in extreme events. Even for those guys, it provides just a small boost. If you're a normal Joe huffing around a track for two or three lunch breaks a week, it's better to focus on powering yourself with a regular diet, including complex carbohydrates, rather than substituting a short-term binge of complex carbs, says Dr. Colgan. A regular diet including complex carbs will steady your insulin level and prevent a fatiguing surge-and-plunge pattern in your blood sugar.

Dependence on simple sugars is woefully rampant in the United States, says Dr.

Colgan. Once, in conjunction with a research project, he sought out a person with hypoglycemia, or very low blood sugar. Knowing that the incidence of hypoglycemia was less than 1 in 100, he screened 120 students with the idea that one genuine case might turn up. Instead, he found that a third of the students had "functional" hypoglycemia—artificially brought on by a diet of pastries and other sweets.

"The students had created a system whereby their bodies could not work without putting simple carbohydrates into them," Dr. Colgan reports. "They ate a doughnut and drank coffee before their first lecture in the morning, and as soon as they got out, they'd have some other processed carbohydrate and stimulant. Then they would go about their business until lunchtime, when they would eat more simple sugar. They created a system where their bodies relied on a trickle of sugar in order to keep their insulin level, and that's very bad.

"A lot of people who think they are fit do the same thing. If we take food away from such individuals, by the end of the day they're shaking—their blood sugar is down, they're in hypoglycemia. Anyone who's fit and healthy and eats the right diet should be able to go 24 hours and still have plenty of energy. Unfortunately, our society breeds people who eat junk food all of the time."

Proteins:
The Original Bodybuilders

If proteins were people, they'd all have answering machines, car phones and chock-full appointment calendars. They are busy little chains of amino acids.

Your body is constantly tearing down

Carbohydrate Sources

Here is the carbohydrate content in grams of commonly consumed foods.

Apple	21
Baked potato	21
Banana	26
Bran flakes, 1 oz.	25
Bread, white, 1 slice	15
Bread, whole-wheat, 1 slice	13
Cheese, Cheddar, 1 oz.	7.2
Corn, canned, 4 oz.	19.8
Cornflakes, 1 oz.	25
Green beans, 4 oz.	10
Hamburger, 3 oz.	0
Milk, 2%, 8 oz.	5
Milk, whole, 8 oz.	4.7
Peach	10
Peanut butter, 2 tbsp.	5.4
Rice, 1 oz.	24
Saltine crackers, 4	7
Shredded Wheat, 1 biscuit	26
Tomato	5.3

and building up tissues, which means it has to destroy and then recreate proteins perpetually. Every four to six days, for instance, you get an entire new intestinal wall.

Pick a reaction in the body, and there's probably a protein enzyme behind it. Proteins carry oxygen in your blood. They slide against each other to make your muscles contract. As photoreceptors, they suck up light for your vision.

"Proteins are the building blocks of practically everything in our bodies," says Dr. Caballero. "Particularly, the skeletal muscle and all of the organs that make us function are made of protein."

Your body recycles. It can make at least 30,000 proteins from the 20 amino acids sloshing around inside you. (If that sounds like a lot, consider how many words we can make from just 26 letters.) When it's time to build new tissue, your body breaks down the protein in the old stuff, releasing amino acids, and then uses those amino acids to make new proteins and new tissue.

Some proteins escape, however. (You do cut your hair, trim your nails and use the bathroom, don't you?) And they need to be replaced. There are nine amino acids that your body just can't make fast enough to keep up with the demands of growth and maintenance. They're called essential amino acids, which means you have to get them from an outside source.

So we eat.

Consider the Source

You might hear talk about the "quality" of proteins. Nutritionists aren't making an aesthetic judgment about your food. They aren't talking about freshness. They aren't even saying a particular food has bad or inferior protein.

"High-quality" or "complete" protein is merely a food that contains enough of the nine essential amino acids to support all of the growth, maintenance and repair jobs going on inside of you. These all-in-one proteins come from animals: eggs, dairy products, meat, poultry and fish.

"That's why, traditionally, animal protein has been considered superior," says Dr. Caballero. "Now, with the concern about animal fat, you have to be careful about how much animal protein you eat. It's difficult, if not impossible, to get animal protein without getting some fat with it—like in a steak, for example. But the beef industry is putting a lot of effort into producing lean and extra-lean meat, and I think in moderation that can provide you with quality protein."

If you're trying to trim fat from your diet, remember this: Even in foods that offer incomplete protein, about a quarter of the amino acids are essential. They just need to be matched up with the missing amino acids to get you hitting on all cylinders. Eating a small amount of animal food with a larger portion of plant food can give you a powerful, lower-fat protein boost. You probably practice this strategy all of the time without realizing it. Ever eat bits of stir-fried beef over rice? A splash of milk on your bran flakes? Egg in a sandwich?

Armed with your knowledge of the protein value of plant food, you can balance out the effects of, say, the occasional tryst with a burger and fries. "You can cheat a little bit," says the University of Puerto Rico's Dr. Michael J. González. "But you have to be fairly consistent. You can say, 'I had some french fries this afternoon, so tonight I'm not going to eat meat. Instead, I'll combine some beans with my vegetables.' You have to be aware of your sources of protein in general."

With a little planning, even a totally vegetarian diet can supply all the protein you need. Man does not live by soy alone, of course. You have to eat a variety of plant foods to cover all the bases, says Dr. Caballero. (This eat-lots-of-different-foods approach, if you've been paying attention, is one of the basic strategies for eating well anyway.) One example: Wheat has sufficient amounts of the essential amino acid methionine, but it's low in lysine. Soybeans are the opposite—loads of lysine and light on the methionine. Eat them both in the same day and you have a complete package.

There's an added benefit to favoring plant protein. You get to eat more food. "If you want to avoid meat," says Dr. Caballero, "you have to eat a larger amount of food because the efficiency of absorption of vegetable protein is slightly less than for animal protein. Just eat plenty of vegetables from different sources and you'll get an adequate amount of protein."

America, the Land of Plenty

Not sure you're getting enough protein? Most likely, you have no need to worry. A survey of more than 50,000 people showed that American men commonly consume as much as 110 grams of protein a day—far more than necessary. Only 2 percent of the American population was getting less than 80 percent of the recommended amount.

"The American diet has excessive protein," says Dr. Caballero. "The human body doesn't have any way to store protein, so if you eat a lot of protein, you are going to eliminate it in the urine. It's not clear whether that's detrimental to health in the long term, but certainly it makes your kidneys work more, because the kidneys have to get rid of all that extra protein."

An international panel of nutrition experts recommends that men should eat at least one-third of a gram of protein for every pound of body weight each day. If you weigh 165 pounds, for example, your safe minimum is about 56 grams of protein. Their recommended level at that weight is slightly higher: 62 grams a day.

Where's the Protein?

Here is the protein content in grams for a typical serving of common foods.

Apple	0.3
Bacon, 3 slices	6
Baked potato	3
Banana	1.1
Bread, white, 1 slice	2
Bread, whole-wheat, 1 slice	3
Cheese, Cheddar, 1 oz.	7
Chicken, 3 oz.	27
Corn, canned, 4 oz.	2.5
Cornflakes, 1 cup	2
Egg, fried, 1 large	6
Green beans, 4 oz.	1
Green peas, 4 oz.	4
Hamburger, 3 oz.	21
Kidney beans, ½ cup	7.5
Milk, whole or 2%, 8 oz.	8
Pork, 3 oz.	23
Tuna, 3 oz.	24
Peanut butter, 2 tbsp.	10
Rice, ½ cup cooked	2
Roast beef, 3 oz.	19
Shredded Wheat, 1 biscuit	3
Tomato	1

Vitamins: The Chemical Alphabet Soup

Vitamins are the diplomatic corps of the body. With a quiet nudge here and a gentle stroke there, their minuscule ranks wield a huge influence over the processes of your body. It's also a sure bet we don't know everything they're up to.

Vitamins are a lively field of research, but there still is a lot to be learned. And wherever you have gaps in scientific information, the void will surely be filled by mystery, intrigue, myths and snake oil salesmen. That means it's particularly important to arm yourself with solid knowledge before deciding, for instance,

whether to take a vitamin or mineral supplement.

We do know that vitamins are substances the body needs in tiny amounts before a host of chemical processes can happen, particularly interactions with enzymes and the release of energy from carbohydrates, protein and fat. They play many other roles, aiding in such things as vision, hormone production and immunity.

Some vitamins also help protect you from the leading men-killer diseases. Beta-carotene (a form of vitamin A) and vitamins C and E have gained a lot of attention for their antioxidant qualities. The natural process of oxidation creates highly excited assassin molecules in your body called free radicals, which are linked to cancer and cardiovascular disease. Antioxidants act as bodyguards. They jump in to get oxidized by the free radicals, limiting the damage to your body.

The Best Source: Food

Nutrition experts say the very best way to get your vitamins is to eat lots of different, wholesome foods—particularly fruits and vegetables. A vitamin pill will supply you with important, but narrowly specified, chemicals. Real food covers the nutritional bases much more thoroughly, not only with vitamins and minerals but also with carbohydrates, protein, fiber and, probably, some crucial substances that haven't even been identified yet.

In 1994 the RDA (Recommended Dietary Allowance) was replaced by the Daily Value—a point of reference for consumers to help show how a specific food fits into a total healthy diet. The Daily Value of a particular food is sometimes the upper limit, or it can be the recommended amount of that particular food.

"I would recommend trying to consume at least five servings of vegetables and fresh fruits every day. There is clear evidence that people who do that have less incidence of a number of diseases," says Dr. Caballero. "There are hundreds of substances we don't know anything about in fruits and vegetables, and a lot of them have antioxidant properties. It is still uncertain which group of them is actually active."

Suppose it's 20 minutes to midnight, you've only had 73 percent of the Daily Value for thiamin, and you're fresh out of pork chops. Nutritional disaster? Relax. Keep in mind that the Daily Values for vitamins are generous—they calculate what your body actually requires, plus a safe amount of padding. Also, Daily Values are not a hard-and-fast dictum that you

must bow to each and every day. Think of them as an average you want to meet over several days.

In special circumstances your diet may fall short of what you need to stay healthy, and you should huddle with your doctor about whether you need a boost from supplements. Maybe you've been dieting long-term, have food allergies, take certain medications, drink alcohol excessively or follow a vegetarian diet. And maybe, despite your best efforts, you've spent too much time in the shadow of the golden arches and you'd like some nutritional insurance.

"Sure you should be able to eat correctly. You should be able to exercise every day, brush your teeth twice a day, floss and do everything right. But nobody does," says Dr. Liz Applegate of *Runner's World* magazine. "We tend to seek out food not for its nutritional value but for its taste and psychological or emotional benefit. Men are also quick to grab something at a fast-food outlet or a convenience store—more for convenience or for the good taste. They're not saying, 'Hey, does this have enough folic acid in it?'

"My approach is to take a multivitamin for insurance, to take one every two to three days. Not so you can say, 'Now my diet's fine,' but just to cover the bases if you do fall short on folic acid. It's found in green, leafy vegetables and citrus fruits, but not a lot of men are eating kale and Swiss chard and broccoli on a regular basis."

How to Take Out Insurance

If you've decided you like working with a net, Dr. Applegate offers these guidelines for buying a multivitamin.

Get the right balance. Find a supplement that provides 100 to 150 percent of the Daily Value for the 13 recognized vitamins (see page 18), plus zinc, selenium and, if possible, copper. It also should contain smaller amounts of iron, calcium and magnesium. Men require less iron than women, and an excess may be linked to heart disease because it's a powerful oxidant. So make sure the iron content is at or below 10 milligrams. Calcium and magnesium should be present at 10 to 25 percent of their Daily Values. The Daily Value for calcium is 1,000 milligrams; for magnesium it is 400 milligrams.

Save your dough. Pass on a supplement that requires you to take three or four doses a day. That's an expensive hassle. Generic brands are generally just as good as the costlier stuff. Timed-release pills and effervescence are expensive gimmicks, and natural or organic sources for vitamins aren't necessarily better, explains Dr. Applegate.

Pass on the extras. Supplements labeled "high potency" or "therapeutic" typically contain excessive doses that may be hazardous. Forgo such nonessential, unproven nutrients as rose hips, "vitamin B_{15}," inositol, PABA, rutin and bioflavonoids, Dr. Applegate says.

Forget megadosing. Many vitamins and minerals become toxic and even deadly in large doses, so a more-is-better philosophy is foolhardy. At the very least you're flushing gold down the toilet, literally and figuratively, since the excess of many vitamins comes out in your urine. But fat-soluble vitamins, like A, D and E, can build up dangerously in your body, Dr. Applegate says. Moderation, then, is the best policy.

How to Get What You Need

In the early 1900s, scientists isolated thiamin ("Hey, this stuff dissolves in water.") and then vitamin A ("Whoa, this one dissolves in fat."). The discoveries created two broad categories for vitamins. It's a handy distinction because the vitamins in each category share a number of properties. Excess fat-soluble vitamins are stored by the body, for instance, while excess water-soluble vitamins tend to be urinated out as waste.

Nutritionists prefer to call some of them by their scientific names (thiamin instead of B_1, for instance), so it helps to be bilingual.

Vital Information

Here are some facts about vitamins we knew you couldn't live without.

- Ever wake up in the middle of the night wondering why there's no vitamin B_4 or vitamin F? Some gaps in the naming sequence were left when vitamins were "discovered" and those discoveries were later declared invalid—the substance was an already-known vitamin or it wasn't a vitamin at all.

- Polar bear liver is so rich in vitamin A, at 600,000 retinol equivalents per 100 grams, that it's considered a toxic source. So skip the polar pâté.

- Some scientists consider vitamin D to be a hormone, not a vitamin, because your body can produce it from sunlight. When you get vitamin D from your food, though, it's technically a vitamin.

- Humans are one of the few mammals that cannot make their own vitamin C and have to get it from food. Bunnies make their own vitamin C, for instance. Ironically, you won't get any vitamin C by eating rabbit meat. Caribou, moose and muskrat meat provide a tiny bit.

- Any vitamin B_{12} in your food is there because microorganisms generated it. In plant food it's only found in poorly washed root vegetables or where bacteria penetrated the roots of legumes. (The best sources are liver, kidney and meat.)

- Your body produces new red blood cells at the rate of at least 200 million per minute. You wouldn't want a vitamin B_{12} deficiency to get in the way of that, would you?

Occasionally, you see the term *equivalent* used. This means the vitamin comes in a few different forms with varying potency, and one form has been chosen as the yardstick by which the others are measured.

If it's not mentioned below, refer to the list on page 29 to determine how much is in one serving of a particular food.

Fat-Soluble Vitamins

Vitamin A

Role: Required for normal vision, reproduction, cell development, growth and immunity. Beta-carotene, chemically related to vitamin A, is an antioxidant.

Major sources: Liver, egg yolks, whole-milk products, cantaloupes, peaches, carrots, cooked spinach, broccoli, tomatoes, lettuce, green peas, green beans, canned corn.

How much men need: The Daily Value is 5,000 international units (IU) (1,000 micrograms RE—retinol equivalents), what you would get by consuming three ounces of tuna, one eight-ounce glass of whole milk, two ounces of Cheddar cheese and one-half cup of cooked spinach.

Vitamin D

Role: Aids absorption of calcium, bone-building and nerve-muscle interaction.

Major sources: Canned sardines, canned salmon, canned herring and fortified foods, like milk.

How much men need: The Daily Value is 400 IU (10 micrograms), what you would get in a quart of fortified milk.

Vitamin E

Role: As an antioxidant, it protects a wide range of chemicals, cells and tissues from oxidation damage.

Major sources: Superfortified cereals (containing added vitamins and minerals), shellfish, greens (mustard, turnip, kale, collards), fried fish, fried potatoes, spaghetti with tomato sauce, chili, peanuts and peanut butter,

chicken dishes and pizza.

How much men need: The Daily Value is 30 IU (20 milligrams α-TE—alpha-tocopherol equivalents), the amount you would get by eating a serving of spaghetti with tomato sauce, coleslaw, greens, fried potatoes and a slice of pie.

Vitamin K

Role: Helps to regulate clotting in the blood.

Major sources: Green leafy vegetables, fruits, tubers, seeds, eggs, dairy products and meats.

How much men need: No Daily Value recommended. The RDA is 80 micrograms. A spear of broccoli will do ya—four times over.

Water-Soluble Vitamins

Vitamin C

Role: Necessary in the bone-building process, the formation of neurotransmitters, the activation of hormones and detoxification processes in the liver. It helps the body use iron, calcium and folic acid. Vitamin C also is an important antioxidant.

Major sources: Oranges, grapefruits, cantaloupes, sweet red peppers, raw spinach, boiled broccoli, fortified cereals.

How much men need: The Daily Value is 60 milligrams, which you would get in a single orange. Optimal dosage is much debated, however, and some researchers advise 250 to 1,000 milligrams a day.

Folic Acid

Role: Required for the growth and division of the cells of all life forms. Fast-growing cells, such as red blood cells, are particularly sensitive to deficiencies.

Major sources: Liver; cold cereals; pinto, navy and other dried beans; spinach; asparagus; seeds; okra and broccoli.

How much men need: The Daily Value is 0.4 milligram (400 micrograms), the amount that you would get by eating one serving of regular cold cereal and a serving each of pinto or navy beans, broccoli and okra.

Cobalamin (B₁₂)

Role: Essential for DNA synthesis and cell division. Red blood cell production is particularly sensitive to deficiencies.

Major sources: Liver, oysters, roast beef, ground beef, bacon, ham, whole milk, fried eggs.

How much men need: The Daily Value is six micrograms, which you would get by consuming six ounces of tuna and two eight-ounce glasses of whole milk.

Pyridoxine (B₆)

Role: Involved in nearly all aspects of protein and amino acid metabolism.

Major sources: Chicken, fish, whole-grain cereals, egg yolks, bananas, avocados, potatoes.

How much men need: The more protein in the diet, the more vitamin B_6 you need. The Daily Value is two milligrams, which you would get by eating a chicken breast, a baked potato and a cup of navy beans.

Thiamin

Role: Involved in the metabolism of carbohydrates.

Major sources: Pork, peas, beans, whole grains, fortified breads.

How much men need: The Daily Value is 1.5 milligrams, which you would get from one serving each of cornflakes, OJ, ham, peas, rice, baked potato and whole-wheat bread.

Riboflavin

Role: Involved in growth and repair of tissues; release of energy from blood sugar, fatty acids and amino acids; production of hormones and formation of red blood cells.

Major sources: Milk, liver, kidney, whole grains, fortified breads, broccoli, asparagus, potatoes, peas and orange juice.

How much men need: The Daily Value is 1.7 milligrams, which you would get by having one serving each of cornflakes, roast beef, milk, low-fat cottage cheese, broccoli and a banana.

Niacin

Role: Essential for the release of energy from carbohydrates, fat, protein and alcohol.

Major sources: Baked goods, cereals, meats, tea, coffee and beer.

How much men need: The Daily Value is 20 milligrams (20 milligrams NE—niacin equivalents), which you would get by consuming one serving each of cornflakes, chicken, whole-wheat bread and canned corn.

Pantothenic Acid (B₅)

Role: Aids in the metabolism of carbohydrates, fat and protein and helps to synthesize hormones, neurotransmitters and other essential compounds.

Major sources: Raw avocados, raw broccoli, bran, organ meats, dry milk and eggs.

How much men need: The Daily Value is 10 milligrams. You could get that by eating two servings each of liver, broccoli, avocados and brown rice.

Biotin

Role: Biotin has a variety of metabolic roles, including the synthesis and oxidation of fatty acids, oxidation of carbohydrates and the metabolizing of several amino acids. It also helps the immune system function.

Major sources: Liver, kidney, peanut butter, egg yolks, yeast, cauliflower, legumes, nuts and cereals.

How much men need: The Daily Value is 0.3 milligram (300 micrograms). You would get that by consuming one serving each of liver, green beans, nuts and oatmeal.

Minerals: The Basic Dirt

In his country music classic "16 Tons" Merle Travis hit on a basic, scientific truth when he noted, "Some people say a man is made out of mud." If it weren't for the "mud" in you, the mineral elements, you wouldn't be much of a man. You count on zinc for sex drive, for instance, calcium for the bones that let you stand tall and magnesium for the muscle action to haul around those 16 tons of coal that Travis wrote about.

Name a bodily process and there's bound to be a mineral involved. Enzymes are behind virtually every chemical reaction in your body, and a third of the known enzymes need mineral ions around before they can do their thing. Non-enzyme proteins make use of minerals, too. Hemoglobin, for example, uses iron ions to bind itself to oxygen, which is carted around your bloodstream by hemoglobin.

While they're crucial to life, the minerals in your body don't amount to much bulk. Pile together all 56 of the minerals known to be in a 165-pound man, and you'd have just enough dirt for a couple of mud pies—less than 7 pounds. There would only be a tenth of an ounce of iron—not nearly enough to make a fist worth singing about.

Scientists say 16 of those minerals—including the ones detailed below—are essential, meaning you couldn't live, grow or reproduce without them. Eleven others, including silicon, nickel, fluoride and tin, are involved somehow in biological reactions.

Mining for Good Health

While Americans typically get an adequate balance of minerals in their food, two minerals are particularly worth keeping an eye on, says Dr. Caballero. "Zinc is linked to spermatogenesis—it's important for development of the gonads," he says. "Although the usual diet can provide the correct amount, this is a nutrient you need to make sure you get enough of. The main source of zinc in the diet is animal meat.

"The other mineral to consider for men is iron. In women the risk with iron is deficiency.

In men it is the opposite. There already are two or three major studies showing that the more iron men have in their blood the more risk they have of heart disease." Iron is thought to oxidize fat in the bloodstream, he says, causing it to cling to artery walls, which leads to arteriosclerosis.

Men should avoid taking iron supplements unless they are taking them under a doctor's supervision, for short periods of time, to treat anemia. It's not likely that you would get excess iron from food.

"The absorption of iron from the intestine is tightly regulated," Dr. Caballero says. "So it's unlikely that you could get too much iron, for example, by eating a lot of beef. It would have to be from taking a lot of supplements on a regular basis, at least for several months."

Here's a rundown of several minerals that are important to your health.

Zinc

Role: Ever hear the expression "That'll put lead in your pencil"? It's not lead that makes your sexual stylus perform, it's zinc. This mineral is important to your sex drive, fertility, wound healing, immunity and the senses of smell and taste.

Major sources: Lean beef, turkey, oysters, cereal, beans and wheat germ.

How much men need: The Daily Value is 15 milligrams, which you would get in a serving of roast beef, a half-cup of oysters, a cup of beans and two eight-ounce glasses of whole milk.

Calcium

Role: Crucial for bone formation and prevention of osteoporosis, blood clotting and neurotransmitter function. By the way, osteoporosis—bones weakened by a lack of calcium—is not just a women's disease. A third of the broken hips related to osteoporosis occur in men.

Major sources: Milk, cheese, yogurt, ice

cream, sardines, almonds, sesame seeds, broccoli, green leafy vegetables and soybeans.

How much men need: The Daily Value is 1,000 milligrams, which you would get in two eight-ounce glasses of skim milk and two servings of broccoli.

Copper

Role: Helps to prevent heart disease and assists T-cells and antibodies in the immune system.

Major sources: Liver, shellfish, nuts, cocoa, mushrooms, whole-grain cereals, gelatin, peas, beans and fruits.

How much men need: The Daily Value is two milligrams a day. Three or four oysters would do it. So would three ounces of Alaskan king crab, a baked potato with the skin and a cup of white beans.

Magnesium

Role: Crucial for muscle activity, conduction of nerve impulses and protection against heart disease.

Major sources: Vegetables, legumes, seafood, nuts and dairy products.

How much men need: The Daily Value is 400 milligrams, which you would get by eating a cup of spinach, two servings of broccoli, an ounce of sunflower seeds and two tablespoons of peanut butter.

Selenium

Role: A component of certain proteins, selenium is particularly known for assisting antioxidant protection.

Major sources: Organ meats, meat, fish, cereals, dairy products, broccoli, cucumbers, onions, garlic, radishes and mushrooms. The more protein in your food, the more selenium you get.

How much men need: No Daily Value. The RDA is 70 micrograms. Three ounces of canned tuna would put you over the top.

Mineral Nuggets

Here are some facts about minerals we knew you couldn't live without.

- You lose 420 micrograms of zinc each time you ejaculate.

- There are 29 minerals floating around in your body for no reason scientists have been able to deduce yet. Those include gold, silver, mercury, aluminum, lead, bismuth, gallium, antimony and lithium.

- Tension, anxiety or grief can interfere with your body's efficiency at absorbing calcium. A study of college men found that their calcium absorption dropped under stressful conditions, like studying for exams.

Iron

Role: Involved in the transportation of oxygen and formation of red blood cells.

Major sources: Liver, meat, fish, poultry, cereal products, apricots, kidney beans, potatoes, peas, raw spinach and raw broccoli.

How much men need: The RDA is 10 milligrams. Three ounces of roast tenderloin, a cup of enriched raisin bran and a baked potato (with the skin) would do the trick. But before you load up your plate, consider: Men hold onto their iron better than women and generally don't need extra. And remember, there's evidence that high iron stores can contribute to heart disease.

Water: Go with the Flow

Like it or not, you're half sloshed. More than 50 percent of your body is H_2O. A lack of the stuff will kill you more quickly than a lack of any other nutrient.

Think of your body as a big, porous water bag. Each day as much as four quarts of water leak out, and each day you top it off with up to four quarts more. This squishy tank comes with an array of regulating equipment—kidneys, lungs, skin and some hormones, for instance.

The captive water inside you is the solvent where most of the life-giving chemical reactions take place. It also serves as a lubricant and a coolant, and it flushes unwanted stuff out of your body.

Under normal circumstances adults should consume about a quart of water for every 1,000 calories in their diet. So if you take in 2,500 calories a day, you need 2½ quarts of water. Only about two-thirds of that comes directly from beverages, though. Solid foods are actually half water, on the average, and that counts toward your daily intake.

"A lot of water is lost in urine and sweat and through respiration," says Dr. Caballero. "Especially in the summer, people have to drink what we call free water—just plain water. And sometimes people don't realize that this is important. I think it's a good idea to have a couple of glasses of water while you are working on hot days. Certainly any soft drink will provide the fluid, but remember that each one of those has 100 calories or more." If plain water bores you, says Dr. Caballero, try the lightly flavored, zero-calorie waters available at many food stores.

Staying well-watered is in your best interest. You sweat out large amounts of water when you work out. Even if you are in good shape, your athletic ability drops if you lose just 3 percent of your body water. And studies show that a 5 percent loss will cost you 20 to 30 percent efficiency on the job. At 10 percent water loss you show symptoms of severe dehydration—nausea, impaired performance, loss of appetite, decreased urination, muscle spasms and increased pulse and respiration—and you run the risk of heart failure. A 20 percent water loss can kill you.

Electrolytes: Only for the Long Run

If you own a jockstrap, you've probably heard of electrolytes. These are a variety of mineral salts—potassium, sodium and chloride are the most important ones—whose ions are dissolved in your body's water. In a complex chemical system this electrolyte orchestra carefully regulates the flow of water inside you.

You commonly lose 1,000 milligrams of sodium a day in your sweat, 2,400 milligrams on a hot day or because of a tough workout. Nevertheless, you generally get all the electrolytes you need from your regular food and drink. The idea of giving athletes salt tablets went out with the slide rule. Modern sports drinks that promise to replace your electrolytes are fine, but salt depletion is really only a problem in ultraendurance events.

"If you do half an hour or even an hour of exercise and sweating, it is very unlikely that you will need any electrolyte replacement," says Dr. Caballero. "But if you are running a marathon, you probably need this type of special replacement."

When you're working out, remember that the sensation of thirst lags behind your body's needs. Before a strenuous session, drink four to six ounces of water and have another drink every 10 to 15 minutes during the workout. Try to drink more than you actually feel like drinking.

When you urinate, check the color. If it's pale, that's good. If it's dark yellow, there's not enough water available to the kidneys, and they're turning out a denser mixture of waste in the water to compensate.

Fiber: The Straight Poop

Pardon the bathroom talk but, frankly, fiber helps you take a good dump, and with that comes a number of important health benefits.

For example:

• A high-fiber diet helps to protect you from cancer of the colon, possibly because it sweeps carcinogens out of the intestines more quickly or because it encourages advantageous chemical reactions in the digestive tract.

• Fiber produces soft, bulky feces, preventing the inflammation that comes with bricklike stools. Researchers from Harvard University and Brigham and Women's Hospital in Boston tracked 48,000 men for four years and found that those who ate lots of fiber in the form of fruits and vegetables were 42 percent less likely to develop diverticular disease than those who got the least fiber.

• It helps to lower cholesterol, leaving you less prone to heart disease.

• While you're consuming foods high in fiber—fruits, vegetables and whole grains—you're usually getting another dietary bonus: complex carbohydrates.

Nutrition experts recommend consuming 20 to 30 grams of fiber a day. Five daily servings of fruits and vegetables and six servings of grains (the less processing the better) will do the trick. American men typically get only 15 grams a day.

"In our country, where we consume a lot of processed food, fiber intake is extremely low," says Dr. Caballero. "Therefore, we have an effort by industry to add back the fiber and by people to consume more unprocessed foods."

Fiber In, Fiber Out

Fiber is indigestible carbohydrate. It sweeps all the way through your digestive system without being absorbed into the body. There are two kinds.

• Insoluble fiber, such as cellulose. This does for your stool what it once did for that squash or carrot you ate: It gives it bulk.

Fiber Options

Here is the dietary fiber content in grams of some common foods.

Apple	2.6
Baked potato	1.4
Banana	1.4
Bran flakes, 1 oz.	8.2
Bread, white, 1 slice	0.8
Bread, whole-wheat, 1 slice	2.4
Corn, canned, 4 oz.	1.3
Cornflakes, 1 oz.	2.8
Green beans, 4 oz.	1.8
Green peas, 4 oz.	5.4
Hamburger, 3 oz.	0
Peanut butter, 2 tbsp.	2.1
Shredded Wheat, 1 biscuit	3

• Soluble fiber, found in fruits, some legumes and grains. This stuff forms a gel that slows the rate at which food passes through the small intestine, thus increasing the absorption of nutrients. It also increases the excretion of bile acids and slows the rate of cholesterol absorption. Some soluble fibers trap bile acids in the gut, according to one theory. The body makes bile acids out of cholesterol, so when soluble fiber escorts them out of the body, the liver has to pull cholesterol from the blood to make more. The result: lower cholesterol.

Dr. Caballero recommends that people increase their fiber intake just by eating the right foods. But if you're having trouble wolfing down that much plant food for some reason, the fiber supplements available in drugstores are a reasonable backup.

"You have to try the supplements and see which one fits," says Dr. Caballero. "Some of those fibers are produced by a fermented bacteria and may produce a lot of gas or even cramps. But there's nothing wrong with them."

Understanding Fat

The Heart of the Matter

It has been reported that when a murderer named Donald Snyder entered Sing Sing, he weighed 150 pounds. He doubled his weight with heaping meals, and even on his last day, the New Yorker was demanding mounds of pork chops and eggs. Snyder's plan: to grow too large for his final seating. Nevertheless, on July 16, 1953, the electric chair still fit him like a warm glove.

A high-fat diet isn't likely to extend your life either.

Sure, you need *some* fat to stay alive. Besides serving as an energy source, it gives structure to every cell in your body. It helps to regulate bodily functions, it insulates you against heat loss and it cushions your vital organs.

But men, on average, get 38 percent of their calories from fat. You don't need nearly that much, and this overconsumption of fat can lead to killer conditions, like heart disease and cancer.

"The national recommendation is to consume no more than 30 percent of your daily calories as fat, but that is sort of a compromise by committee," explains Johns Hopkins University's Dr. Benjamin Caballero. "There is nothing magic about 30 percent. I think 20 to 25 percent is reachable without being a Tibetan monk.

"A few fats are essential for us, but you can fulfill all those needs with a little over 5 percent fat in your diet. A diet completely free of fat is not healthy, but you have a very wide margin between 5 and 30 percent."

The Mammoth Appetite

Thog, your Cro-Magnon grandpa 35,000 years removed, feasted on bison, reindeer, horse and mammoth. When he gobbled down meat, his body wisely stored any excess fat to get him through lean times.

"Evolutionarily, we were prepared to have these periods of starvation, ready to survive. That's why we accumulate fat so easily," says the University of Puerto Rico's Dr. Michael J. González. "As my nutritionist friends say, the problem today is the refrigerator. We used to go search and hunt for food and now we just open the refrigerator. Calories are very accessible."

For Thog, fat was a conveniently dense energy source—nine calories per gram. Carbohydrate and protein provide only four calories per gram. Unfortunately, Thog's modern descendants have inherited bodies programmed to railroad excess fat right to the waistline. Chemically, the fat you eat is pretty much in ready-to-store form, and it takes minimal effort for your body to sock it away. Your body is able to convert excess protein and carbohydrate into storable fat, but that process requires extra energy.

A Chokehold on Your Heart

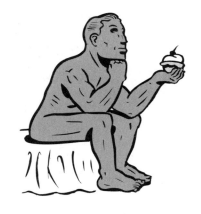

Excess fat in the diet may throw your body out of whack in several serious ways, contributing to heart disease, high cholesterol, obesity, diabetes and some cancers. Saturated fat (the stuff found in meat, poultry and dairy products) and trans fats (found in margarine and shortening) seem to be the most dangerous kinds.

Coronary heart disease is the leading cause of death in the United States and other affluent countries. Much of it is traceable to saturated fat, which raises the level of LDL ("bad" cholesterol) in the blood. LDL leaves fatty deposits in the coronary blood vessels. Narrowed blood vessels leading to the heart can cause a heart attack. Strokes can be caused by narrowed blood vessels leading to the brain.

In a program called the Seven Countries Study, scientists tracked 12,763 middle-aged men for 25 years. The more saturated fat and trans fats the men consumed, the more likely they were to die of coronary heart disease. For instance, the men in Tanushimaru, Japan, received just 3.8 percent of their energy from saturated fat and had a 4.5 percent death rate from heart disease. On the other extreme, the men in east Finland received 22.7 percent of their energy from saturated fat and had more than six times the Japanese death rate from heart disease: 28.8 percent.

Scientists generally agree that monounsaturated fat (like olive oil) and polyunsaturated fat (like corn oil) are much more heart-friendly than saturated fat. Those fats either have no effect on—or they lower—your blood cholesterol. But which is more beneficial? Christopher Gardner, Ph.D., who studies disease prevention at Stanford University, combined the results of 14 cholesterol studies done in the last decade. The resulting overview surprised him: It's a tie—they're equally beneficial to your cholesterol.

"We were stunned, because we expected it to be one way or the other," says Dr. Gardner. "They were really virtually equivalent." This doesn't mean the two oils are equal in all respects, he notes. Polyunsaturated fatty acids, like sunflower or safflower oil, might encourage tumor growth.

Fat in Your Food

Here is the total fat content in grams of some common foods.

Apple pie, (⅛ of a 9-inch pie)	13.8
Bagel, plain, 1	1.1
Beef frankfurter, 1	12.8
Cheese, Monterey Jack, 1 oz.	8.5
Chocolate chip cookie, store-bought, 1 small	2.3
Cornflakes cereal, 1 cup	0
Cottage cheese, 1%, ¼ cup	0.6
Croissant, butter, 1 medium	12.0
Doughnut, plain, 1 medium	10.8
Egg, scrambled	7.3
Ice cream, regular vanilla, ½ cup	7.2
Milk, 1%, 1 cup	2.6
Milk chocolate, 1.55 oz. bar	13.5
Peanut butter, 2 tbsp.	16.0
Pork sausage, smoked, grilled, 1 link	21.6
Sandwich, ham and cheese	15.5
Sandwich, roast beef	13.8
Spaghetti, cooked, 1 cup	0.9

Corralling Cholesterol

Good cholesterol, bad cholesterol. Sounds like a B western being played out in your bloodstream. Fine—go buy a white hat. You have the lead role.

Your body actually needs some cholesterol, but it makes a sufficient amount all on its own. The extra cholesterol you get from food is just icing on your arteries. When doctors test your blood, they measure the cholesterol in terms of milligrams per deciliter. This is the famous "count" for total cholesterol, which is best kept under 200. Almost half of all Americans fall on the dangerous side of that figure.

To get a really meaningful measure of your health status, make sure your cholesterol test gives a breakdown for HDL and LDL. Your count for the harmful LDL should be below

130. For the protective HDL, you want a count above 35. An HDL count below 35 could mean danger even if your *total* cholesterol appears to be safe at or below the 200 mark.

Cholesterol is only found in animal food: meat, fish, eggs and dairy products. In food there's no good or bad cholesterol. That issue only applies to how your body transports cholesterol once it's in your body (HDL ushers it out of your body, LDL paints it on the walls of your blood vessels).

Identifying the cholesterol in your food is not hard. In general, the same foods that are high in saturated fat are also high in cholesterol—beef, ice cream and béarnaise sauce, for instance. So a low-fat approach to eating will also cut your cholesterol consumption. Eggs and seafood are exceptions: While they are low in fat, they have more cholesterol, ounce for ounce, than any other food.

So aside from eating low-fat, what can you do to lower cholesterol? Scientists offer these suggestions.

Feast on fiber. Studies show that eating foods that are high in soluble fiber helps to lower your cholesterol, even for people who are already on a low-fat diet. Doctors say adding three grams per day of oat fiber, for example, can lower your total cholesterol level by five to six points. So order up the beans, whole-wheat pasta, oat and wheat bran cereals, fruits, like apples and oranges (eat the white stuff under the peel, too), and just about any vegetable.

Grab a grapefruit. Antioxidant vitamins are on your side in preventing heart disease. Government researchers say men who get lots of vitamin C, for instance, have elevated HDL levels. (Go for the citrus fruits and juices.) In Finland, researchers found that arteries clogged more slowly in men with high LDL levels when they got lots of beta-carotene (car-

The Fat Budget Made Easy

If you want to be totally fastidious about tracking your fat intake, you'd better hire an accountant and a nutritionist to follow you around with one of those little food scales. But here's an easy way of tallying it all in your head—without the entourage.

In the table shown here, find the fat limit that's appropriate for your weight. This figure represents 20 percent of the calories a guy your size would typically consume in a day, says Robert Kushner, M.D., director of the nutrition and weight control clinic at the University of Chicago. Eat more, and you're destined to gain body fat. Eat less, and you'll lose.

Anytime you fix something to eat, check the nutrition label. Look at the serving size and look at the amount of fat

rots and sweet potatoes) and vitamin E (wheat germ and mangoes).

Hit the bricks. If you're overweight, dropping excess poundage is essential to controlling your cholesterol, doctors say. A one-two punch of weight loss and exercise will lower total cholesterol, reduce the level of triglycerides in your blood, raise the HDL level, reduce blood pressure and reduce the risk of diabetes. And when you weigh less, your dietary efforts—paring out the saturated fat and dietary cholesterol—do a better job of lowering your LDL. To lose weight, try moderate aerobic exercise, like jogging or cycling, for 30 minutes per session four or more days a week.

The Fat-Cancer Link

Dietary fat has been linked to colorectal cancer, prostate cancer, pancreatic cancer and breast cancer, among others—even lung cancer in each serving. If you're eating, say, twice the serving size listed, you'll have to double the amount of fat listed. In your head keep a running total of the fat you consume. When you're done putting things in your mouth for the day, check your actual total against your limit.

Easy, huh? Now send your accountant home. Tell him you might have a job for him next April.

Pounds	Fat Limit (g.)
130	40
140	44
150	46
160	49
170	53
180	55
190	60
200	62

in nonsmokers. Scientists aren't sure whether a high-fat diet directly creates cancer tumors, but there's strong evidence that a steady diet of some fats will grease the skids for tumors that do appear.

Dr. González says animal studies demonstrate that omega-6 fatty acids (corn oil) promote tumor growth, while omega-3 fatty acids (fish oil) slow tumor growth.

"Let's say we had a 20 percent corn oil diet," he says. "You would have tumor growth that was very high. If you had 15 percent corn oil and 5 percent fish oil, the tumors would grow but they would grow less. And as you increase the fish oil, they would keep decreasing in size."

It's tough to say how much of that applies to people, Dr. González says. You can't do such experiments on humans, and our complex metabolisms and varied diets cloud the issue still further.

But cutting back on fat overall is a good

cancer-fighting move, he says. "There's no good fat, just as there's no sweet lemon, like my grandmother used to say. If I had to use one, I'd rather use olive oil. About half the studies show that it doesn't enhance tumor growth. In other studies it enhances, but it never enhances as much as corn oil."

By now, you're clamoring for advice for trimming fat out of your diet and your body. Let's cut to the chase.

Treat your meat. When you buy beef, go for the lean stuff: USDA Choice or Select. Prime meats have more marbling and, therefore, more fat. Lean meat doesn't have to be tough. When you soak beef in a marinade, acids tenderize the meat and add taste. Try citrus juice and herbs, low-sodium soy sauce, vinegar or yogurt. And here's a no-brainer: Organ and lunchmeats are high in fat, so avoid brains, hearts, kidneys, livers, sweetbreads (that's the thymus gland of an animal), bologna, hot dogs and sausages.

Read the package. Check the nutrition and ingredients labels on food packages before you buy. In a split second you can find out the total fat and saturated fat content.

Eat early. Consume at least 60 percent of your calories in the morning. Even if you made no changes in your diet and exercise, this move would trim fat from your frame, according to A. Scott Connelly, M.D., a California researcher specializing in nutrition and metabolism. In the evening the excess blood sugar in your system is more likely to be converted into body fat.

Bake to shake fat. If you gravitate toward fruits, vegetables and grain foods, you'll automatically sidestep a good amount of fat lurking out there. But keep an eye on the chef. A baked spud, for example, is virtually fat-free (unless you smear it with butter), but you'll get 11 grams of fat in just 14 french fries.

Read before You Eat

How to Profit from the Pyramid

Glance at the Food Guide Pyramid on the opposite page. Does your vision go blurry? Does your mind drift, sleepily reminded of fourth-grade textbook illustrations?

Well, smack yourself sharply across the jaw and give it another look. You've probably been ignoring a tool that's as simple as a paper clip, as versatile as a Swiss Army knife and as intuitively accessible as a Macintosh computer.

While we're at it, have you ever looked at the Nutrition Facts panel that appears on almost every food item you buy? No? That's worth two smacks, because you've really been asleep.

The point is that a lot of the information you need to make wise food choices is right under your nose. It's clear and it's reliable. Even those brightly lettered health claims on food packages have to follow U.S. government guidelines. What you may have been dismissing as hype or inconsequential fine print can help you stay healthy, gain energy and manage your weight. All you need to do is engage your brain.

"Nutrition labels list nutrients that play a role in chronic disease. The levels of these nutrients have public health significance," says Carole Adler, R.D., a dietitian in the Food and Drug Administration's (FDA) Office of Food Labeling. "I think if men understood that, they would feel more inclined to read them."

So here's how to navigate the Food Guide Pyramid and food label, including the Nutrition Facts panel. If you master both of these, we'll stop

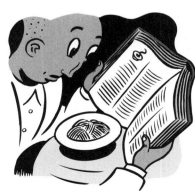

making you slap yourself. People are starting to stare, you know.

How the Pyramid Stacks Up

The Food Guide Pyramid is a dietary cheat sheet, a visual guide reminding you of three concepts in one glance.

- Variety: Eat lots of different stuff, hitting all the food groups.
- Moderation: Watch your serving sizes, and go easy on the fats, oils and sweets.
- Proportion: Notice how big a block the grain and pasta group gets on the pyramid? Load up on those foods. See how much smaller the dairy group is? A little dab'll do ya.

The pyramid's sections incorporate the five major food groups as defined by the United States Department of Agriculture. Sorry, the tip of the pyramid—reserved for soft drinks, candy, butter, oil and the like—doesn't rate major food group status. The second tier from the top comes mostly from animals. These foods—like milk, meat, fish and eggs—are big sources of protein, calcium, iron and zinc. The third tier is plant food, fruits and vegetables, which is high in vitamins, minerals and fiber. Grain foods make up the foundation of the pyramid, providing complex carbohydrates, vitamins, minerals and fiber.

"The idea is to guide people in balancing amounts of certain products versus others," says the University of Puerto Rico's Dr. Michael J. González.

Check out the number of servings a day listed for each food group. Men are supposed to gravitate toward the high end of the range, particularly if they're active. Does 11 servings of grain sound like a belly-buster of an eating plan? Maybe not, if you consider what counts for a serving: one slice of bread, one ounce of cold cereal or half a cup of cooked cereal, rice or pasta. The servings add up quickly: If you eat cereal and a slice of toast at breakfast, a sandwich at lunch, a cup of pasta at dinner and three or four small, plain crackers for a snack, you're at seven servings already.

Here's what counts for a serving in the other food groups.

- Vegetables: 1 cup of raw, leafy veggies; ½ cup of other vegetables, cooked or chopped raw; or ¾ cup of vegetable juice
- Fruits: a medium apple, banana or orange; ½ cup of chopped, cooked or canned fruit; or ¾ cup of fruit juice
- Dairy foods: 1 cup of milk or yogurt; 1½ ounces of natural cheese; or 2 ounces of processed cheese
- Meats: 2 to 3 ounces of cooked lean meat, poultry or fish; ½ cup of cooked dry beans; 1 egg; or 2 tablespoons of peanut butter

The food guide's illustrations are a helpful touch, Dr. González says. It's no coincidence that broccoli appears, for example. High in vitamins and fiber, "it's almost the perfect food," he says.

Speaking of illustrations, most folks don't notice those tiny circles and triangles sprinkled over the pyramid. They represent the fat (circles) and added sugar (triangles) that appear in various foods. The more fat and sugar a food group is likely to have, the more little circles and triangles you'll see in that section of the pyramid.

What's in This Stuff, Anyway?

If the Food Guide Pyramid is your overall battle plan, then the Nutrition Facts panel is your ammunition in the trenches.

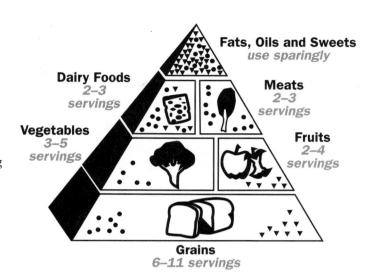

Fats, Oils and Sweets
use sparingly

Dairy Foods
2–3 servings

Meats
2–3 servings

Vegetables
3–5 servings

Fruits
2–4 servings

Grains
6–11 servings

Okay, the trenches look an awful lot like grocery aisles, and you're lugging granola bars instead of grenades. But this is where the nutritional battle is won or lost—the moment when you decide whether to toss an item into your cart or to leave it on the shelf.

When you're considering buying a packaged food, turn the item around until you find that little box with the words "Nutrition Facts" at the top. For most foods, the FDA requires manufacturers to list the amounts of 13 nutrients and calories from fat, and it allows the voluntary listing of ten additional dietary components. If you want to ponder as many as 23 nutrients for every food item you buy, be our guest. Just don't forget to take your laptop computer, and turn off the lights when you leave the supermarket. In the real world you're more likely to zero in on the handful of items on the nutrition label that most concern you.

"It really depends on what your goals are," Adler says. "Let's say you're a man trying to focus on weight management and a low-fat diet. Then you may want to look at the information on calories, calories from fat, total fat, saturated fat and cholesterol. Of course, if your doctor says you're sodium sensitive and you're trying to lower your blood pressure, then you would also focus on the amount of sodium in the product."

Suppose you're looking for a snack cracker and you pull a box of chili-and-cheese-flavored Munch 'ems off the shelf. You see at the top of the chart that a single serving is 28 crackers. (This serving size is not a recommendation—it's just what the FDA says is an amount customarily consumed in one sitting.) If you eat twice that many when you snack on crackers, then you need to double all of the nutrient amounts you find on the chart.

But let's assume you're a 28-cracker snacker. If you're concerned about calories and fat, you check out these figures next: 140 calories, 35 of them from fat. A quick calculation tells you that this food gets 25 percent of its calories from fat. You're trying to keep your fat consumption to less than 30 percent of calories, so these Munch 'ems won't throw you seriously off track, if you've kept your fat intake in check during the rest of the day.

You also see that there is a total of four grams of fat in a serving and beside that figure is the notation "6%." That percentage is what's called a Daily Value, which gives you an idea of how this snack fits into your overall eating plan. A serving of these crackers will give you 6 percent of the maximum amount of fat you should be eating in a day for a 2,000-calorie diet. So you make the call: How's that jibe with whatever else you want to eat? How do these crackers stand up nutritionally against other snacks?

Two important points about those Daily Values. First, they're based on the assumption that you consume 2,000 calories a day, which is low for lots of men. Generally speaking, a guy who's 5 feet 11 inches tall, medium-framed and moderately active needs about 2,750 calories a day. Second, for troublesome nutrients, like fat, cholesterol and sodium, consider 100 percent of the Daily Value to be a maximum, a mark you

Why a Pyramid?

Remember *The $100,000 Pyramid* game show? Not to be outdone, the federal government spent nearly $1 million on test marketing the Food Guide Pyramid before introducing it in 1992. Among the other hot contenders were a jigsaw design (which test subjects found puzzling), a circular pie chart (which reminded kids of pizza) and a grocery cart filled with paper sacks of varying size (they bagged it—too ambiguous).

"A couple of things make the pyramid work. For one thing, it's very simple. Also, it's not a new shape," says Dan D. Snyder of the communications company Porter/ Novelli. Snyder was the designer on the case when the United States Department of Agriculture commissioned a new food guide in the late 1980s. "Everybody knows what a triangle looks like, so it's not trying to teach a consumer a new shape, like a shopping basket or a fruit bowl."

The Food Guide Pyramid first took shape on Snyder's sketch pad as he watched a focus group from behind a two-

want to come under. For user-friendly stuff, like carbohydrates and dietary fiber, think of the Daily Value as a minimum, a target you want to hit or surpass.

Judging a Food by Its Cover

One reason you pulled that box of crackers off the shelf was the inviting phrase " . . . but with 33% less fat than regular tortilla chips." Hmmm, sounds good. But years of dubious nutrition advertising claims have left you with a powerful knee-jerk cynicism. The fact is, health and nutrient claims on food packages are now closely regulated. Knowing the rules that manufacturers have to play by will make you a more confident shopper.

"There used to be consumer confusion,"

way mirror. He and a government staffer were toying with block shapes that represented different food groups when they decided to stack the blocks to form a triangle.

That pyramid is now a cultural icon. Sixty-three percent of Americans are familiar with it, according to a *Parade* magazine survey, and 57 percent of those people say they obey its recommendations an average of four times a week.

If you're among its followers, remember this about the pyramid's design: Higher is not better. "The things that you should eat the most are at the lower part," notes the University of Puerto Rico's Dr. Michael J. González. "Sometimes people will say, 'Hey, why are grains down low when we should be eating more? They should be up there.' "

Snyder says an upside-down pyramid was actually tested, but "people thought it was not stable. It looked like it was going to fall over." Besides, the name "Food Guide Yield-Sign-Shape" doesn't have the same ring to it.

says Adler. "A firm would state on the label that a food product was low-fat, and the firm itself would make that determination with its own definition. Now those definitions are provided by the FDA, so they have to be accurate."

Here's how the FDA defines some of the most common terms found on food packages.

- Free: Contains none, or only a trivial amount, of the nutrient named. "Fat-free," for example, means that there's less than half a gram of fat per serving.
- Low: You can eat this food frequently without blowing your limit for the nutrient named. "Low-fat" means three grams of fat or less per serving, for example.
- Lean and extra lean: These terms describe the fat content of meat. Gener-

ally speaking, "lean" means fewer than 10 grams of fat per serving (and per 100 grams). "Extra lean" means fewer than 5 grams of fat per serving (and per 100 grams).

- High: Contains 20 percent or more of the Daily Value for the nutrient named.
- Good source: A notch below "high." Contains 10 to 19 percent of the Daily Value.
- Reduced: Somebody's monkeyed with this food to get at least 25 percent less of a nutrient or calories than the regular product.
- Less: Contains 25 percent less of a nutrient or calories than some similar food we'd like to point an accusing finger at. (See the tortilla chip claim mentioned previously.)
- Light: A third of the calories or half the fat has been booted out of this food. Or, for a food that's already low-calorie and low-fat, half the sodium has been removed. Careful: Packages may still use the word "light" when speaking of color, as in "light brown sugar."
- More: Contains at least 10 percent of the Daily Value of a nutrient above what's in the regular version of the food. For example, if a regular juice contains 34 percent of the Daily Value of vitamin C, then the high-test version claiming "more" vitamin C must have at least 44 percent.

Food packages also are allowed to carry statements associating nutrition and prevention of specific diseases. Examples: calcium and osteoporosis and fiber and cancer. Such a statement might read, "While many factors affect heart disease, diets low in saturated fat and cholesterol may reduce the risk of this disease." Foods carrying these reminders generally have to contain significant amounts of the nutrient being touted.

Buying Cookbooks

Read between the Lines

In the kitchen you want to be known as a chowder hero, not a chowderhead. The cookbook you use is a key player in your culinary success, so before you shell out clams for one, choose carefully.

Ever find yourself staring numbly at a store's monolithic, floor-to-ceiling display of cookbooks? To start the selection process, consider the different categories of cookbooks, says Jonathan A. Zearfoss, a certified executive chef who teaches advanced cooking at The Culinary Institute of America in Hyde Park, New York.

• Encyclopedic cookbooks: These large volumes are a valuable part of your collection. Roughly half recipes of traditional and "homestyle" cooking and half explanation of cooking techniques, they aim to educate. Examples: *Mastering the Art of French Cooking* by Julia Child, Simone Beck and Louisette Bertholle, *James Beard's American Cookery* and *Joy of Cooking* by Irma S. Rombauer.

• Broadly themed cookbooks: Books that address a large subject, like Mediterranean cuisine, are a good bet. They tend to involve many different cooking techniques and a great variety of recipes.

• Single-subject cookbooks: If you have a passion for flat breads, Tunisian cooking or some other narrowly defined subject, go ahead and buy these. Such books are great for rounding out a collection. But if your cookbook cupboard is bare, start out with a more broadly focused book. "Nobody's going to eat Tunisian every day," Zearfoss

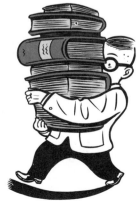

says, "although you might eat in the Mediterranean style more than once a week."

• Restaurant cookbooks: Fun but dicey. "A lot of times restaurant cookbooks are interesting, especially if you've been to the restaurant," says Zearfoss. "But take a good look at whether those recipes are really adapted for the home cook, because a lot of times they're straight from the restaurant and hard for people to execute."

• Coffee-table cookbooks: Beautiful but limited. "The photographs are usually very attractive but probably near impossible to recreate," Zearfoss says, "so they will no doubt cause frustration. The recipes tend to be abbreviated and not give really specific instructions."

You can cover all the bases with eight or ten cookbooks, Zearfoss says. Aside from encyclopedic texts, "You would need one on baking, maybe one on breads and pastas and a couple on 'hot' areas of cuisine such as Mediterranean, Asian and Mexican. I think you would impress people by knowing a little about those."

Check the Fine Print

Keep that credit card safely tucked in your wallet for a few more minutes. Before you buy a cookbook, make sure it's authoritative, health-oriented and will actually see lots of action in your kitchen. Here's how to make sure of those things.

Review résumés. Find an "About the Author" passage in the cookbook you're thinking of buying. Consider the writer's professional training and length of experience. For books about ethnic cuisines, has the author traveled in the originating country to get that extra degree of authenticity? Remember that the term "master chef" is used loosely on cookbook jackets. If the initials C.M.C. appear after the author's name, that's an industry-recognized professional qualification: certified master chef.

Strike the right match. Even the best cookbook by the culinary genius of the century will do you no good if you aren't turned on by the food it helps you create. "Flip through the recipes and ask yourself, 'Are these the kinds of foods I'd like to be eating?' You need to match a book to your taste buds," says Evelyn Tribole, R.D., a consulting nutritionist in Beverly Hills, California, and author of *Healthy Homestyle Cooking* and *Eating on the Run*. "Ask yourself if these are the kinds of ingredients you have ready access to. If you don't mind shopping for special ingredients, that's fine. Figure out, in terms of your style of cooking, if it's the kind of stuff that you like to do."

Think ethnic. Gravitate toward cuisines that have a built-in emphasis toward low-fat, high-carbohydrate foods such as fruits, vegetables, beans and whole grains. "Mediterranean cooking and Asian cooking are hot not only because people like them but they also already contain the elements of healthful cooking," Zearfoss says. "Particularly foods from the Pacific Rim—Vietnam, Thailand and Japan."

Sample the Recipes

The dirty little secret of recipes is that they're an inexact science. No written instructions can tell you exactly how to chop an onion, for instance. And if an author attempted to, you'd never read your way through it all. Besides, no two onions are alike, no two cooks are alike and no two kitchens are equipped in the same way.

This means that the author of a recipe has to make assumptions about the reader, and you may or may not be that audience. If a cookbook's recipes are not useful to you, all you have bought is a very expensive doorstop. So here are some points to consider when

> ## The Lean-Living Library
>
> Here are more cookbooks that will help you explore the joys of luscious and lean cooking.
>
> - *Healthy Homestyle Cooking* by Evelyn Tribole
> - *Prevention's Cooking for Good Health*, edited by Jean Rogers
> - *American Heart Association Cookbook*, fifth edition, the American Heart Association
> - *Jane Brody's Good Food Gourmet* by Jane Brody
> - *Jacques Pépin's Simple and Healthy Cooking* by Jacques Pépin

sizing up the recipes in a cookbook.

Go long. A long passage of instructions in a recipe does not mean it will rival the Manhattan Project in complexity. The text may just be helpful detail about a cooking technique. "For tomatoes one recipe might say 'peeled, seeded and chopped,' whereas a more detailed cookbook might tell you *how* to peel, seed and chop a tomato," says Zearfoss.

Run an equipment check. Scan a couple of recipes and note the tools necessary for each preparation. A cookbook gets more and more expensive each time it requires you to trot over to a cooking store to buy new gear.

Test for success. In the better cookbooks all recipes have been worked up in a test kitchen to make sure measurements and directions are accurate. Look for mention of testing procedures in the foreword.

Sweat the details. Your dinner guests arrive in 20 minutes and you're feeling pretty smug—until you get to the last line of the recipe for your main course: "Simmer for four hours." To help you schedule yourself in the kitchen, look for cookbooks that highlight preparation and cooking times. Also, recipes that list nutritional breakdowns—the calories, fat, fiber, cholesterol and sodium in each serving—take a lot of guesswork out of your nutritional decision making.

Staying Motivated

Eat from the Tree of Knowledge

A funny thing happens when you start reading about nutrition. An extra apple finds its way into your lunch bag. Frozen yogurt shoulders your usual carton of ice cream aside and scrambles into your shopping cart. The mayonnaise jar gets lost in some back corner of the fridge as you reach repeatedly for the mustard instead.

Your mind absorbs the knowledge of how to feed your body well, and the behavior follows. Why? For one thing, when you peel away some of the mystery surrounding a subject, mastering it does not seem nearly so great a task.

"When it is all brand new to you, there is a learning curve. So you need to be prepared to give yourself that," says nutritionist Evelyn Tribole. "But when you get more comfortable with it, eating nutritiously isn't so daunting. When you say 'changing your lifestyle,' it sounds like such a tall order, but it doesn't have to be a big deal. When you first get started, you think, 'Oh, the food is going to taste bad,' or 'I have to take more time.' But this is not true at all. It is healthy eating and it tastes fabulous and it doesn't have to take any more time."

When you learn about nutrition, you're addressing the root of some of your own body's problems. If you try to change your eating patterns without that underpinning of knowledge, you're setting yourself up for failure.

So read, read, read about food. Immerse yourself in the science. It will not only inspire you to improve your eating, but it will arm you with ideas about how to best develop a program that meets *your* needs. To heck with those one-size-fits-all diet plans. A weight-loss study, for instance, showed that people who devise their own programs do a better job of slimming down and keeping the fat off than people who are prescribed a specific eating approach.

Winning the Mind Game

As you begin to master the art of eating, expect to stub your toe against gender roles now and then. Rest assured there is nothing inherent in being a man that precludes you from becoming food-fluent—society just set up a few obstacles. How many guys in your high school, for example, took home economics?

"Men, in terms of their gender role around food, haven't been very oriented toward nutrition. They have been more oriented toward tastes, fun, satiety and things like that," says Cornell University's Dr. Jeffery Sobal. "It is not a biological thing. It is a gender role. Women are more tied to the food system, from buying food, to preparing food, to making sure that food gets eaten right."

You're going to discover that eating well is addictive. "I have people really look at how they are feeling," Tribole says. "Like, how did it feel today that you ate consistently and you didn't skip meals? Is your energy level different? Is your ability to concentrate on work different?

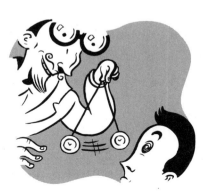

Often you will see a real benefit. When you know those benefits and you feel them, they become self-perpetuating—motivating."

Dean Ornish, M.D., reported similar motivation among his heart patients. He conducted groundbreaking studies that showed heart disease could be reversed in patients who followed diets that are extremely low in fat. In his book *Eat More, Weigh Less*, Dr. Ornish tells of a distinguished Japanese physician who collared him at an international scientific meeting. "Dr. Ornish," he asked, "do you brainwash your patients in order to get them to change their diets and lifestyles?"

The answer is no, of course. But Dr. Ornish did learn these things about motivation from patients who participated in his studies: Making wholesale changes in diet can actually be easier than taking small steps, because you feel better more quickly. And the joy of feeling good is more motivating than fear of disease or death far down the road.

Tools of the Trade

Here's more advice from nutrition experts on how to keep yourself motivated to eat well.

Fear no food. Chocolate bars, eggplant, cheeseburgers, yogurt. They're all just things. There are no devils hiding in some foods and angels residing in others. There are no "bad" foods or "good" foods. If you insist on binding your emotions to these inanimate objects, you're on the path to perpetual frustration and, possibly, eating disorders. That's giving these little lumps of nutrients far more power than they deserve. When you understand food, *you* hold the power.

Imagine success. Spend some time every day visualizing yourself meeting your nutritional goals. If you need to eat more fruit, picture yourself rinsing grapes in the morning and placing them on a dish at the breakfast table. See yourself ripping a banana off the bunch on the kitchen counter and tossing it into your briefcase for an afternoon snack.

Work on small goals. Long-term goals,

Got the News Blues?

The breathless television announcer flashes onto the screen: "You won't *believe* what food they're now saying is bad for you! News at 11!"

It's easy to feel like your whole lifestyle is under attack. One day they say movie popcorn will choke your heart. The next day it's kung pao chicken, and then it's lasagna.

If healthy eating boils down to tofu and rice cakes, you say, who needs it?

We posed that question to the source of many such news reports, Jayne Hurley of the Center for Science in the Public Interest.

Relax, she says. Information is a tool, not an enemy.

"We're not telling people what to eat," Hurley says. "I read some of these editorials and I think some people depict me as waving a finger in people's faces saying, 'You can eat this, you can't eat that.'

"That's not the point. If you want to eat something that's full of fat, you should know it. How else are you going to adjust the rest of your diet unless you really know what's in it?"

---

like losing four inches around the waist, can be intimidating. You'll find short-term achievements more inspiring, something you can accomplish the same day—maybe substituting an apple for the cookie you usually eat for an afternoon snack. After all, success at a long-term goal requires an accumulation of smaller victories. Tribole calls this approach "living in the moment."

"Broadly sketched, people think eating well is important—they say, 'Oh yes, it really counts.' But where they get caught is in the moment, specific situations—*that* is where it really counts," Tribole says. "It is consistency over time that is going to make the difference. It is not going to be some new magic bullet or some new magic diet. It is how you can implement your eating approach consistently."

Be forgiving. Every man is seduced by the occasional chocolate fudge brownie. Don't torment yourself with guilt. What's important is how your eating pattern averages out over the weeks and months. If you don't loosen up and allow the occasional indulgence, you'll get frustrated and give up altogether.

Record the pros and cons. Draw a line down the middle of a sheet of paper. On the left side write all of the reasons for sticking to your eating plan (feeling better, your belly's flatter, better health). In the right column write all of the costs of sticking to your program (fewer beers and hamburgers, less freedom to pig out). Now you have a visual representation of the motivating thoughts and the negative thoughts swirling around this business of managing your nutrition. Post the list. Being open about your negative feelings and reminding yourself of the positive aspects will help to keep you motivated.

Chart your progress. Keep a weekly record of your weight and the time you spend exercising. Also track your cholesterol count, blood pressure and other indicators whenever you have them checked. Look back over the record periodically to remind yourself of your progress.

Keep a food diary. Devise a way to keep track of exactly what you are eating every day. Depending on what most concerns you, you might write down the fat and sodium content of each item. At first, don't even try to make any changes. Nutrition experts say that just keeping track of what you eat motivates

---

Shifting into Gear

Having a little trouble transforming your new nutritional knowledge into action? Here's a three-step breakdown of the motivational process that may help.

- **Set a goal. Goals focus your efforts. Make them reasonable and specific. For instance, "Within a month, I will be eating beans in at least four meals a week."**
- **Vary the pattern. Variety will keep you interested. Get those beans in a soup one day, a salad the next and in chili the day after that.**
- **Reward yourself. When you meet the goal, celebrate. Go to a movie *you* want to see, not some ho-hum flick you had to negotiate with your significant other. Or buy a new pair of sunglasses. Or a music CD. Whatever makes the accomplishment feel special and seals the deal in your mind.**

---

you to make better choices.

Try teamwork. When you're trying to change eating patterns, it's tough to go it alone. Even tougher if your house is a swamp of negative influences. A two-year study examined men who were put on a cholesterol-lowering diet. When their wives were supportive—without nagging—the odds of meeting their goals were up to five times better. So make food a togetherness thing: Shop, cook and eat together.

Don't forget exercise. If you're trying to lose pounds, managing your diet is only part of the equation. Just about all weight-control programs require you to move your body around more to burn calories. But you don't have to suddenly start training like an Olympic athlete. Say you weigh 154 pounds. If you played tennis for just 15 minutes a day, you'd burn 9 pounds of fat within a year. And if that sounds like a long time to wait, well, remember that patience really is rewarded: Scientists say that pounds lost gradually are more likely to stay off than pounds lost quickly (more than one or two pounds a week).

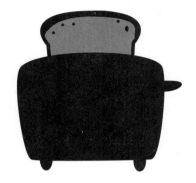

Part Two

Eating at Home

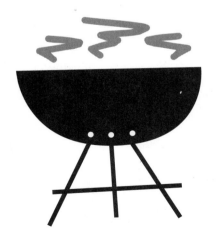

A Man's Kitchen

Tools You Need to Do the Job Right

Junu Kim grew up with his mother's admonition ringing in his ears: "If a man steps into the kitchen, his testicles will fall off."

Now in his thirties, Kim is married and does most of the cooking. And fortunately for Kim and millions of other modern men, it turns out his mom was wrong. "Both of those boys are still there," Kim says proudly.

It all leads us to wonder where this idea came from that a man's castle stops at the kitchen door. Kitchens are full of guy stuff. And we're not just talking about the beer and leftover pizza in the fridge. The kitchen is the place where lettuce gets slammed against the countertop, the place where huge, sharp knives dismember chickens and turkeys. And it's the place where slabs of meat are beaten with wooden hammers. Indeed, in many ways a man's kitchen is a toolshop in disguise. Some comparisons:

Workshop	Kitchen
saw	chef's knife
X-acto knife	paring knife
pliers	tongs
T square	measuring cup
workbench	cutting board
table saw	food processor

Just like the workshop, you need to choose your kitchen equipment carefully. Here's what you need to outfit a man's kitchen.

Going under the Knife

Enter the world of kitchen knives. You have your fillet knife, your butter knife, your boning knife and your bread knife. Then there's your ham knife. And the cook's knife. A carving knife. An oyster knife.

Seems like they make a different knife for every cutting job around. But you only need two: a big chef's knife for chopping and pulverizing and a smaller paring knife for whittling and dissecting. What you need to look for:

Steel yourself for action. If you can find a carbon steel knife, you're in business. That's the best kind of knife around. But it also rusts easily and is hard to come by, says Annemarie Colbin, founder of the Natural Gourmet Cookery School in New York City and author of *Food and Healing* and *The Natural Gourmet.* To prevent rust, wash it and dry it immediately after each use.

Stainless steel is also a good buy. It will need more sharpening than a carbon steel knife, so you'll have to buy a sharpener as well. If you're the kind of guy who lets dishes and utensils pile up in the sink until you run out of clean ones, it might prove to be a wise investment.

Look for rivets. Rivets are those small, flat circles you see in the knife's handle. Think of them as screws that hold the blade to the handle. A good knife has at least two rivets on each side, Colbin says.

Better check your tang. If you look down at the handle, you can see where the blade runs through the middle of it. That's called the tang. The best knives are called full tang, which means the steel goes all the way to the end of the handle. A half-tang, where the steel goes halfway down the handle, is much better than no tang. If you buy a knife without rivets and without a tang, expect it to fall apart.

Make it resin-ate. The handle should be treated with resin so it's smooth and waterproof.

Be ready to pay. You'll have to fork out a lot of dough

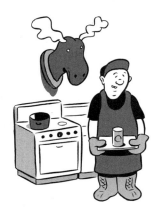

to buy a good set of kitchen knives. They can run more than $200, but if you demand quality, they're the top of the line. *Consumer Reports* rated kitchen knives and chose J. A. Henckels Four Star, J. A. Henckels Professional "S," and the Cuisine de France Sabatier as the top three lines. Just a chef's knife from any of those companies might cost close to $100. If you just want a good, inexpensive knife, *Consumer Reports* rates Ekco Best Results Professional as tops. A four-piece set will run you only about $30.

Stay sharp. Once you get your knives, you'll want to keep them sharp. "Knives that are dull will slide and therefore can hurt you more easily," Colbin says. "Most people think it's the other way around."

Your knife is dull when:

- It slides a lot when cutting.
- It makes cracking sounds when cutting. Knives should be quiet.
- You run it lightly across a tomato and it doesn't break the skin.

If your knives are really dull—we're talking about going back and forth over the tomato four or five times with no result—you should get them sharpened professionally, Colbin says. Look under "Sharpening Service" in the phone book.

You could try to do the job yourself with an oilstone or diamond-impregnated block, both of which are sharpening tools that can be found where you buy knives or in some hardware stores. The process requires lots of patience. There are also electric sharpeners that will fix super dull knives.

The idea, though, is to keep your knives from getting that dull, and that means sharpening them every time you use them. So when you buy your knives, you should also get a sharpening steel from the same company. Hold the blade at a 20-degree angle against the steel and draw the blade across the steel from

---

Something's Burning

Firefighters call it CWI—cooking while intoxicated. "We have a lot of those calls in New York City," says Joseph Bonanno, Jr., a fireman with Ladder Company 152 and author of the *Healthy Firehouse Cookbook*. "You come home after partying with your friends and say, 'Oh, man, I gotta get something to eat.' You put something in the oven. You sit on the couch. You fall asleep." Next thing you know, someone's banging on your door and there's smoke pouring out of the kitchen. The half-dozen firemen waiting there are not amused. And all you can do is feel stupid and mutter, "That damn pizza I put in the oven."

---

handle to tip. Do that three or four times on each side of the blade before each use.

Some knives come with holders that will sharpen your knives for you. Every time you pull out or put back the knife, the blade drags across a sharpening mechanism. But be wary. *Consumer Reports* warns that many of the samples they tested did not function properly.

Be an Iron Man

You'll need pots (deep containers you can boil water in) and pans (shallow containers you can make pancakes in) of at least four different sizes, says Colbin.

- A one- to four-quart pot
- A huge six- to eight-quart stock pot
- A ten-inch skillet (with deep sides)
- A seven- to ten-inch sauté pan (with shallow sides)

If you have a big family or just tend to use every burner on the stove when you cook, you'll want some additional pots and pans in various other sizes. You're looking for stuff that's easy to clean and hard to break. Here's what to look for.

Get a good conductor. No, not the kind who comes in tails waving a baton. You need pots and pans that conduct heat evenly so that you won't burn as much food. The best heat conductor is silver, but unless your last name is Trump or Forbes, you can't afford that (more than $2,000 a pan). Copper also conducts heat well, but it's easily damaged, is a major-league pain to clean and can release copper into your food, says Colbin. What's left? Aluminum. Because aluminum can make food smell funky, you want the aluminum sandwiched between some other metal, preferably stainless steel—it's easy to clean.

Work out with iron. A cast-iron skillet should last a lifetime. It adds crunch to foods and blackens catfish extremely well. You don't have much sticking and you'll boost your iron intake, says Colbin, because some of it gets in your food. It's also versatile, working equally well on the stove or in the oven, and it's easy to clean, too.

But cooking with cast iron is a workout. The typical cast-iron pan can weigh about three times as much as the typical stainless steel one.

Also, you'll need to season a new one and keep it seasoned to prevent rust. A completely seasoned cast-iron pan takes several months of continuous use and proper care. After that, the pan turns a dark color, possibly black. But you can get great results from a just-seasoned pan. Once you remove the label and the adhesive underneath the label, pour a half-cup of vegetable oil into a 12-inch skillet (use less for a smaller pan) and use a paper towel to spread it evenly over the surface (the sides, too), making sure to rub the oil in well. Pour off the excess

Good Gadgets

There's this device Black and Decker sells that makes waffles that look like kids' building blocks, the kind with letters and numbers inscribed on them. No joke. The waffles come out letters on one side, numbers on the other so your kids can learn to count and say part of the alphabet while they eat breakfast.

Which brings us to the world of gadgets, a place packed with electric carrot peelers, cordless can openers and travel mug coffeemakers. Gadgets are, in sales lingo, things that are supposed to save us time and energy. But we know what they really are: power tools for the kitchen.

But kitchens are only so big, and even the most creative space saver of a guy can't fit every gadget there is to buy in his kitchen. So we did an informal office survey. We wanted to know which ones people bought and actually used and which ones collected cobwebs and rust under the kitchen sink. What follows is a list of gadgets that received a universal thumbs-up.

• Steamer. By now you know steamed food means low-fat food. Steamers cook food quickly without added fat and with minimal nutrient loss. You could steam the food yourself by boiling water and placing a bamboo steamer basket, metal colander or a wire basket above it. Or you could buy an electric steamer. You chop up the food, throw it in, set the timer and wait. Some even cook rice. All you

oil, leaving a thin film on all the surfaces, and bake the pan at 300°F for an hour. Then turn the oven off but leave the skillet inside for a few more hours, preferably overnight, says Tom Ney, food editor for *Prevention* magazine. After that, put the pan on a stove burner and heat it for five minutes on medium high. Let it cool. It's now seasoned.

Don't be a stickler for cost. If cast iron seems like too much work, then go for have to do is put the rice bowl attachment into the machine and follow a few simple instructions.

• **Juicer.** Nutritionists are telling you to drink lots of juice to help you increase your fruit and vegetable servings. This gadget lets you mix up your own concoction. They do come with one problem, according to users: They are hard to clean.

• **Coffee grinder.** Some are so elaborate, you can tell them how finely to grind the stuff—extra fine for espresso, medium for auto drip and coarse for French press. Others are just those simple stainless-steel-bladed, it-does-the-job kind. You can also use it for chopping nuts and spices. Don't buy one unless you're really a java junkie. Otherwise, you'll eventually revert to the preground, store-bought variety, buyers say.

• **Wok.** Buy a nonstick one to cut down on the oil you use. If used properly, it allows for fast cooking with minimal oil. For stir-frying, an electric wok has a slight advantage over a traditional one because you can set a definite temperature. Most cooks, though, may prefer traditional woks. Even over an electric range, the traditional variety can reach the extremely high temperatures essential for wok cookery. Electric woks may have an edge in convenience, but if you want the insanely hot temperatures needed for true wok cooking, you'll probably be happier with the traditional kind.

You can cook an even healthier meal by using chicken stock, vegetable stock, vinegar or wine instead of oil. If you want to use oil, try a nonstick cooking spray. Just be careful to only coat the pan. Don't drench it.

spoons or metal spatulas with it.

Get a grip. Pots and pans come with wooden, plastic and metal handles, and each material has its strengths and weaknesses. Metal handles get really hot, but a pan with a metal handle can be used for baking as well as stovetop cooking. Wooden handles are sturdy and attractive, but you can't put them in the dishwasher if you want them to continue to look nice. *Consumer Reports* pushes plastic handles. Though they aren't as handsome, they are dishwasher-safe, rugged and can usually withstand oven temperatures up to 300°F.

Everything but the Kitchen Sink

You could spend your weekly paycheck on a lot of unnecessary kitchen stuff you'll probably never use, or you could buy what you really need and use the money you save for a weekend getaway for two to a romantic bed-and-breakfast (breakfast optional). It's up to you. Here's what you need.

• Cutting board. Get a big, maple butcher block. "It looks better, it smells better and it lasts longer," Colbin says. How big of a block you buy depends on the size of your kitchen. It should be at least an inch thick and measure at least 12 inches by 24 inches. Which is safer, wood or plastic? Despite some research that gives the safety edge to wood, the jury is still out at this point. Mona R. Sutnick, R.D., Ed.D., a nutrition consultant and spokesperson for the American Dietetic Association, says the real issue is keeping whichever material you use for a cutting board very clean.

• Food processor or blender. Look for a small, inexpensive one that's easy to clean. Use either appliance to puree or chop. A

either stainless steel or a pan with a nonstick coating. Fancy nonstick pans can run you close to $100, and they're not indestructible. If you're a freshman cook, Nancy D. Berkoff, R.D., a culinary instructor at the Los Angeles Trade Technical College, suggests buying the cheapest nonstick pan possible. After all, odds are you're going to destroy it. Once you've learned to be gentle, then you can advance to the more expensive kinds. Just remember not to use metal blender will also mix drinks and crush ice, and you can use the blender to make a cream soup without the cream. Any starchy vegetable or grain such as potatoes, carrots or oatmeal will create a creamy texture in the blender, says Colbin.

• Mixing bowls. Look for something easy to clean that can go from the fridge to the oven and back to the fridge without exploding. Stainless steel bowls are the best, in Colbin's opinion, because they are the lightest and most durable, but they can't go into the microwave like glass or plastic.

• Tongs. You want a pair that fits your hand comfortably and is sturdy enough to pick up an ear of corn without snapping in two.

• Ladle. Make sure it's man-size. It should be big enough to dish out chili a serving at a time.

• Mixing spoons. Think about what you look for in a paint stirrer. That's right: wood. You want wooden spoons for the same reason you want wooden cutting boards. They look better and they are easy to clean. "Also, the wooden spoons last forever. The plastic ones react badly to heat," Colbin says.

• Peeler. The kind that works best, according to Colbin, has the blade sandwiched into the handle.

• Grater. Instead of nicking your knuckles on the rectangular kind, you can buy the circular kind with a hand crank.

• Spatula. For scraping goop out of bowls, buy rubber on a wooden stick. "All of the plastic ones disintegrate. They get really weird," Colbin says. "They get very sticky and disgusting after a short time. Rubber lasts the longest."

Some other things you'll want: garlic press, metal spatula for flipping pancakes, lemon juicer, whisk, strainer, can opener and a hand beater.

Keeping It Cold

Refrigeration and freezing allow us to store food for a long time, but not forever. Assuming you have your refrigerator set at 40°F and your freezer at 0°F, here's how long you can keep some common items.

Food	Refrigerator	Freezer
Eggs, fresh, in shell	3 weeks	Do not freeze
Egg yolks and whites	2–4 days	1 year
Eggs, hard-boiled	1 week	Do not freeze
Liquid egg substitute, unopened	10 days	1 year
Liquid egg substitute, opened	3 days	Do not freeze
Mayonnaise	2 months	Do not freeze
TV dinner, unopened	Do not refrigerate	3–4 months
Soups and stews	3–4 days	2–3 months
Burger/stew meats	1–2 days	3–4 months
Ground turkey, veal, pork or lamb	1–2 days	3–4 months
Hot dogs, unopened	2 weeks	1–2 months, in freezer wrap

Mapping Out Your Kitchen

She's coming for dinner tonight. The one you met in the grocery store olive oil aisle. You lured her to your place by boasting about your culinary skills. Now you're sautéing shrimp, mixing up chocolate mousse and slicing strawberries. She will arrive in less than half an hour and where are the (expletive deleted) measuring cups? You tear the place apart. In your blind frustration you fling open the freezer door. It happens. Measuring cups are sometimes in the freezer. Wham. A pound of ground beef lands on your foot.

Miss Olive Oil arrives at your front door, and you have a broken toe. A little disorganized, are we?

Not to fear. Here's a seven-step program

Food	Refrigerator	Freezer
Hot dogs, opened	1 week	1–2 months, in freezer wrap
Lunchmeat, unopened	2 weeks	1–2 months, in freezer wrap
Lunchmeat, opened	3–5 days	1–2 months, in freezer wrap
Bacon	7 days	1 month
Raw sausage	1–2 days	1–2 months
Smoked breakfast links or patties	7 days	1–2 months
Canned ham	6–9 months	Do not freeze
Whole cooked ham	7 days	1–2 months
Sliced cooked ham	3–4 days	1–2 months
Beefsteaks	3–5 days	6–12 months
Pork chops	3–5 days	4–6 months
Lamb chops	3–5 days	6–9 months
Beef roasts	3–5 days	6–12 months
Lamb roasts	3–5 days	6–9 months
Meat leftovers	3–4 days	2–3 months
Whole chicken	1–2 days	1 year
Chicken pieces	1–2 days	9 months
Fried chicken	3–4 days	4 months

that any clutteraholic can follow.

1. Organize around the stove. "You want to have things within easy reach," Colbin says. "Whatever you use the most should be closest to you." So keep your two knives, your cutting board, maybe a mixing bowl, your pan and your pot near the stove. Think about what else you usually need and put them in plain view. A few exceptions: oils and spices. Nix the wall spice racks. Spices should be stored in darkness. Ditto for oil.

2. Only buy as many appliances as will fit on the counter. Thanks to modern ingenuity, you can get creative about where you put them. Just about everything can be mounted to a cabinet. "If you don't have the space, you have to keep it underneath the counter. A lot of people don't want to take the time to get it

out and plug it in," says Jennifer Anderson, nutrition consultant and spa dietitian at Bonaventure Spa and Fitness Resort in Fort Lauderdale, Florida. "It sounds silly, but you don't want to go past all of your other appliances, pots, pans and mixing bowls and drag it out."

3. Ask for help. Any department store carries an array of organizational helpers. One kitchen helper looks like a circular plastic or wooden rack. You can hang your measuring spoons and cups, a can opener and some other stuff on the sides and stick your mixing spoons, spatulas and other stuff in the center. "I find that to be pretty handy because when I'm cooking, the measuring spoons are right there and they are all together," Anderson says. "It's not like they're mixed up in the drawers and I can't find my quarter-teaspoon."

4. Get a drawer separator. It has slots for your forks, knives and so forth.

5. Keep like things together. Make a breakfast section, a starch section for lunch and dinner and a canned food section. Putting your cereals, oatmeal, oat bran and other morning eats together allows you to go to one place to figure out what you want for breakfast. "Everything's right there so you're not looking all over your kitchen and thinking, 'Oh, nothing looks good in this cabinet, let me try another cabinet,'" Anderson says.

6. In the freezer, keep meat, poultry and fish on the bottom. That way, if some juices accidentally escape, they won't contaminate anything else that's not going to be cooked at a high temperature. Keep the frozen vegetables on top.

7. In the freezer and refrigerator, use the door shelves to stack small items that will easily get lost in the depths.

Seafood

Getting in Tune with Neptune

It's dinnertime and Mr. and Mrs. Blandmouth find themselves in a large but strange East Coast city. They're in town from Nebraska for the Regis Philbin Charisma Conference, and now they need to eat. They're in a daring mood, so they decide on the city's famed seafood restaurant.

As the waiter talks about the sweet pompano, the juicy shad and the rich bluefish, their eyes widen, a slight haze forming over the pupils. Mr. Blandmouth's right pupil wanders to the corner of his eye and catches Mrs. Blandmouth's left pupil in the corner of her eye—a small but inescapable signal that daring is now kaput. "I'll have the baked flounder without the sauce," says Mr. Blandmouth. "I'll have what he's having," follows Mrs. Blandmouth.

The Blandmouths have just ordered a bland meal. "Those who aren't fish eaters, they order plain flounder. I always think it won't have any taste. I guess they have it to say they ate fish," says Richard Bookbinder, owner of Bookbinder's Seafood House 15th Street, a well-known Philadelphia seafood establishment that occasionally entertains visitors like Mr. and Mrs. Blandmouth.

Fishing for Good Health

Fish restaurant and market owners know only too well that seafood can be a hard thing to get to know, but there are many reasons why you should acquaint yourself.

For one, it's a healthy

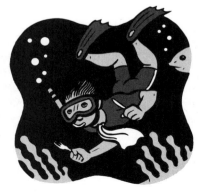

way to get protein and trace nutrients found in beef without also getting the fat and cholesterol. Like meat, fish contains all of your essential amino acids. You only need to eat three ounces of fish every other day to satisfy your daily protein needs. Fish also is a good source of certain B vitamins, which you can't always get from plants.

Seafood usually contains only 5 to 10 percent fat, compared to red meat, which is 30 to 40 percent fat. The leanest of beef—broiled top round—has 4.9 grams of fat per 3.5-ounce serving, compared to the leanest of fish—cod or flounder—which has no more than 2 grams of fat per 3.5-ounce serving.

"Even when you eat what is called a fatty fish, like salmon, it only runs between 6 and 10 percent fat. When you consider a Big Mac is 45 percent fat and french fries are about the same percentage of fat, you're really eating a low-fat diet no matter how much fish you consume," says Gary J. Nelson, Ph.D., a research chemist with the U.S. Department of Agriculture Western Human Nutrition Research Center in San Francisco.

And even seafood that's considered to be high in cholesterol is better than eating meat, Dr. Nelson says. Crab, shrimp and lobster may be higher in cholesterol than other seafood, but their total fat is only between 1 and 2 percent.

"As long as you're not eating it in hollandaise sauce or pan fried in gobs of butter, as long as you're just eating the boiled shrimp, it's so low in fat you're probably better off than eating something else, like cheese or beef or pork," Dr. Nelson says.

Also, the cholesterol in shellfish doesn't come close to what you'll get from eggs. Two eggs at breakfast gives you more than 400 milligrams of cholesterol—100 milligrams more than your daily recommended maximum amount. A 3.5-ounce serving of shrimp (about nine small shrimp) has just 166 milligrams of cholesterol.

Another reason to eat fish perhaps isn't as important as we once thought. For years doctors pushed fish consumption because of an oil called omega-3 fatty acids that was thought to prevent heart disease, arthritis, stroke and diabetes. But researchers have found that fish oil has fewer healthy powers than was formerly believed. It's not a reason to forgo fish, although you can save some money by skipping the fish oil pills. It's just that fish doesn't seem to do anything magical for our hearts.

One study found that increasing your fish consumption from one time a week to every day will not significantly reduce your risk of heart disease. Another found increased fish consumption didn't decrease the risk of heart disease or stroke.

"It seems like they are not the panacea that was hoped for," says Walter C. Willett, M.D., Dr.P.H., professor of epidemiology and nutrition and chairman of the Department of Nutrition at the Harvard School of Public Health and a co-author of both studies. "It's important to remember that you can get omega-3's from plants as well. And there is some suggestion that getting them from plants might be beneficial from the standpoint of heart disease. So I don't think the final answer is in on all forms of omega-3's."

Shellfish Safety

There is truly no bad seafood when it comes to fat and protein, Dr. Nelson says. But you may need to be wary of particular kinds for pollution reasons and if you're allergic.

Shellfish often live amidst the garbage dumps of the sea. Oysters and clams feed by filtering 15 to 20 gallons of water per day, soaking up food particles as well as harmful bacteria and pollutants. Crabs, if they can't find any fresh food, are likely to be scavengers,

eating dead material on the ocean's floor. Both eating habits make the creatures more susceptible to picking up people-sickening germs. It's more an issue with mollusks, like clams, mussels and oysters, because you're eating the entire body—including the stomach. When you eat crabs, you tend to pick out the white meat and stay away from the entrails.

That said, you don't have to give up shellfish. You just need to ask questions when you buy it.

Find out where it came from and whether those waters are clean or polluted, says Doris Hicks, a seafood technology specialist with the University of Delaware Sea Grant Program in Lewes. Each bushel of oysters, clams or mussels must have a tag that is dated and lists where it came from. You can find out about fish safety and other seafood topics by calling the Food and Drug Administration's Seafood Hotline at 1-800-FDA-4010.

Here are two other safe shellfish strategies to keep in mind.

Make sure they open. If the clamshell doesn't open when you cook it, you should throw the creature away. The closed shell means the clam inside wasn't subjected to enough heat to kill the bacteria that are naturally present.

Don't get a raw deal. Think of downing raw oysters as bungee jumping. It can be a great experience, and it can be a deadly one. You can prevent raw oyster problems by not taking a chance and avoiding raw seafood altogether, says Hicks. Also, if you don't know where your oysters came from, not eating them during the months between May and August may help you avoid a rare type of food poisoning caused by red plankton.

If you have a chronic disease (such as liver, kidney, gastrointestinal), you should never eat raw oysters or any raw shellfish, because you are more susceptible to its bacteria. The same rule applies to those suffering from immune-suppressing diseases such as AIDS or tuberculosis.

What You Need to Know

Now we're back to Mr. and Mrs. Blandmouth. Had they been a tiny bit more daring, they could have ordered grilled swordfish or tuna—both good starter fish. Neither have bones. They come in thick steaks, and they have more flavor than flounder. At least Mr. and Mrs. Blandmouth could have gone home to Nebraska boasting about their dinner and their auto-graphed photo of Regis Philbin to their neighbors.

For the Mr. and Mrs. Blandmouths everywhere, here's a basic guide to fish.

• The bonehead variety. Most restaurants will debone your fish, so you usually won't have to worry about taking little bites and then using your tongue to smush the meat around in search of throat-scratching bones. But some fish are really boney. And if you don't like pulling food from your mouth every once in a while, they are best eaten carefully. These include trout, shad, sea bass and catfish. "You would almost have to be a brain surgeon to get all the bones out," Bookbinder says.

• The robust variety. If you wake up the day after and your dog is still licking your fingers, you had a robust fish. We're talking about the ones with the strong flavor and smell. They are oily with either a pink to red meat color or a blue to gray meat color. These include salmon, shad, tuna, mackerel, mahimahi, bluefish and pompano.

• The "almost like meat" variety. These come in steaks and can be grilled. They are white-fleshed, so they aren't fishy tasting. These include cod, halibut, mako, shark, skate, monk-fish (medallions) and swordfish.

• The pale-faced, flaky variety. These come in fillets and are soft-fleshed and mild tasting. They include orange roughy, perch,

A Burger to Go

By now, we know in our hearts that we can't have all-beef patties—even if we hold the special sauce and cheese—as much as we may want.

But what's the alternative?

Try ground fish.

Fish burgers come in several varieties, including salmon, tuna and, in the summer, Louisiana or Black Drum redfish. A betting man would lay down $100 that fish burgers would flop. And a betting man would lose.

"It caught on right away, especially with the fish-eating vegetarians," says Robert Perose of Perose Seafood in Allentown, Pennsylvania, one of a growing number of stores where fish burgers are sold. "We make it into sausage. We make it into a veal Parmesan. Anything you would use ground beef for, this can be substituted. . . . It's the closest thing to meat you can get."

pollock, catfish, hake, sea trout, tilapia, fluke, flounder and sole.

When you order fish at a fish store, be less concerned about the actual name of the fish than the type. Let's say you're looking for something to grill. Then don't go in and just look at the tuna. Consider swordfish and shark as well, says Hicks. For one, the store might not have tuna that day. Also, allowing yourself to substitute one fish for another can save you money. For instance, though swordfish is avail-able year-round, it's much less prevalent on the East Coast in October and November when fishing is a little tougher because of rough seas and stormy weather. So the price will probably be higher.

Here are some other pointers when buying and ordering fish.

Ask for directions. Let the store owner

Whether you get a salmon burger or a redfish burger, you're doing your heart some good. Both are low in fat. Salmon has less than a gram, and redfish contains less fat than boneless, skinless white chicken meat.

Because they are low in fat, the fish cook much faster than a regular beef burger. It takes about four minutes per side to grill.

We would never recommend that you eat something we haven't at least sampled ourselves, so we had lunch at Perose Seafood one day and tried the Cajun redfish burger. Now, we wouldn't exactly say it tastes like a hamburger. It actually tastes *better* than most burgers. Light and spicy. Juicy. It was a lip-licking meal.

The ground salmon has a stronger fish taste. If you like salmon, you'll like a salmon burger. If you don't like salmon, you won't like a salmon burger.

explain the best way to cook the fish. Many fish store owners don't mind helping you out. Richard and Robert Perose of Perose Seafood in Allentown, Pennsylvania, will even do the work for you. On some nights they sell already prepared fish. For instance, they'll have salmon with honey mustard already smeared on top. A sticker on the box explains how long to bake it. The brothers also have pre-made, microwaveable fish dinners. A chunk of seasoned fish comes with some vegetables and potatoes. Cooking time is only a couple of minutes.

Turn up the volume. Look for a store that handles a lot of fish. That means the fish will come and go quickly. It won't lay around.

Get fresh. You want to get the freshest fish possible. A fresh whole fish will have bright, clear eyes, shiny skin with a metallic luster, bright red gills and smooth, well-attached scales, says Hicks. Also, the flesh should be firm and elastic. It should spring back after you press it.

Fillets should be moist and firm with no dried-out edges or gaping holes. And mollusks—oysters, clams and mussels—should have tightly closed shells. If the shell is slightly open, tap it. If it closes, the creature is alive and edible. If it doesn't move, throw it away.

Keep it cold. When picking out fish at the store, make sure it's cold to the touch. Fish is kind of like ice cream. You want to get it home before it melts, so make your trip to the fish store your last errand. And if you know the drive home in 90-degree heat will last more than a half-hour, bring a cooler or ask them to pack the fish with a bag of ice. At home put the wrapped fish in a bowl and cover it with a bag of crushed ice and store it in the coldest part of your refrigerator, the meat or middle drawer (because it's protected from temperature fluctuations when you open and close the refrigerator door). Uncooked fish should be used within one to two days of purchase and kept between 33° and 34°F, says Hicks. "You want to keep your fish cold but not frozen," adds Perose.

Suffocate and freeze. When freezing fish, you don't want air to get to the fish. Make sure the plastic wrap is skintight, then put the fish in a freezer storage bag or plastic container. This will prevent any damage to the fish from shuffling or rough handling, says Hicks. Fish will keep between three and six months in the freezer depending on the type. Low-fat fish keep longer than fattier fish.

Listen to old Ben. In *Poor Richard's Almanac* Ben Franklin said fish and guests smell after three days. That's how long your cooked leftovers will keep in the fridge, says Hicks.

Meats

Prime Choices for Lean Living

Lucky Fred Flintstone. Sure, he had to settle for Wilma instead of Betty, but when he pedaled home from work each night, he knew he had a steaming, ten-pound slab of brontosaurus steak waiting on his plate for dinner. And just think: None of those doctors who harp on how too much red meat clogs your arteries were even born yet.

Americans eat an average of around 235 pounds of meat a year. "That's an all-time high," says Jens Knutson, director of Regulatory and Industrial Affairs at the American Meat Institute in Washington, D.C. More than half of the meat we consume is red meat. Poultry is next at about 40 percent and fish lags far behind at roughly 6 percent, reports the American Meat Institute.

That old mastodon masticator Fred Flintstone probably wouldn't see anything wrong with those figures, but most doctors would. And while there has been a slow shift from red meat to poultry in recent years, it appears some nutrition-conscious consumers may be counting their chickens for the wrong reasons.

Our Beef Is with Fat

Thanks to advances in food technology, red meat has grown increasingly lean. And researchers have found that our blood cholesterol couldn't care less whether we eat chicken or beef. The meat just has to be lean.

Two studies have pointed to the fat content of beef—and not necessarily beef

itself—as the problem. One study looked at 38 men with high blood cholesterol levels. The researchers found it didn't matter whether the men ate lean beef or lean chicken. Both meats decreased blood cholesterol levels by the same amount.

Another study looked at whether beef protein or beef fat was the cholesterol-raising culprit. The conclusion: the fat.

So as long as it's lean, we can eat as much as we want? Not so fast. There's still cholesterol in the meat to worry about, and most of the cholesterol is in the meat's lean parts. Also, there's the iron factor. One three-ounce serving gives you from 20 to 30 percent of your Recommended Dietary Allowance of iron. High doses of iron have been linked to heart disease.

"The kind of iron you get in meat is particularly troublesome because your body can't regulate its storage," says Harvard University's Dr. Walter C. Willett. By contrast, if you have enough iron from vegetables or vitamin supplements, any excess doesn't get stored, he says.

High red meat consumption also has been linked to colon cancer, the second-leading cause of death from malignancies in the United States.

Still, you don't have to deny yourself the meat you love. You can eat it and still be healthy if you follow some nutritional advice, says Lynne W. Scott, R.D, director of the diet modification clinic at Baylor College of Medicine in Houston. Eat small portions. Eat lean cuts. And eat it along with other low-fat foods.

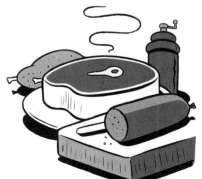

The Kindest Cut

There are really two big things to look for if you want to continue eating red meat and still keep your heart running smoothly: portion size and fat content. Here are some ways to enjoy meat and good health.

Don't gamble with big portions. You can eat up to six ounces of lean meat a day and still be healthy, says Scott. How much is that? Next time you're playing poker with the boys, check out the deck of cards before you deal. That's about the size of three ounces of meat. Then, bet the house that you'll reduce your daily meat consumption to no more than two decks of lean meat a day. Better yet, go ahead and bet your life, because that's what you're really doing.

The stakes are that high. You already heard about cancer. You already heard about iron and cholesterol. But there's yet another reason to eat meat in small amounts: protein. About 15 percent of the calories in your diet should be protein, says the USDA's Dr. Gary J. Nelson. If you're eating 2,500 calories a day, you'll need 300 to 400 calories of protein. Three ounces will more than satisfy that.

"People don't need any more than that," says Dr. Nelson. "In certain cases, excess protein can lead to gout or, much more commonly, kidney stones. If you ate three ounces of fish or beef every other day, you would have no trouble at all satisfying your need for protein."

Select wisely. Many companies will pay the government to grade their meat. Grades are based on the animal's age and the amount of fat in its meat. Beef is graded prime, choice, select, standard, commercial, utility, cutter and canner. You really only need to worry about choice and select. Prime, which contains more marbling of fat in the meat than most of us wish to buy, is usually sold only to restaurants. Choice and select are the grades most frequently found at supermarket meat counters. The others are so tough you'd never eat them as a steak. They are either used in ground beef or in processed meats. Prime tenderloin gets 48 percent of its calories from fat. The same steak rated choice gets 44 percent and select checks in at 39 percent.

Buy lean cuts. In any animal the leanest meat is located where the animal has larger, more active and powerful muscles. This makes sense. Think about your own body. Your biceps are probably much leaner than your rump. We could give you an anatomy lesson for each farm animal, but instead, we'll make it simple. Just look for round, ham and leg cuts, suggests the USDA Agricultural Marketing Service.

When we're talking birds, light meat is lower in fat than dark meat. Backs and the legs have the highest amount of fat.

Read the labels. In general, chicken and turkey are leaner than beef, but you really need to compare the fat content. Some ground beef is leaner than ground turkey. That's mainly because ground turkey can contain skin and fat that drives up the fat content. The same goes for hot dogs. (To be fair, there are some brands of low-fat and fat-free wieners out there, too.) Look at the grams of fat per ounce.

Learning to Love Lean

You know what happens when you cook lean meat. It tastes like lean meat—dry and chewy. It robs your mouth of saliva. It's the ultimate letdown. Here you've smelled steak. You've seen steak. But you didn't really taste steak. When you got done eating, you were still craving steak.

It doesn't have to be that way. Stanley Lobel, a fourth-generation butcher at Lobel's Meats on Madison Avenue in New York City, knows how you feel. And he says there's a really easy solution to the lean steak problem: Marinate it.

Don't worry. You don't have to be Julia Child to pull this off. All you need is a bottle of fat-free Italian dressing, says Lobel, who runs the butcher shop with his brother Leon, son Mark and nephew Evan. Pour it over the steak, then put the steak in the fridge for anywhere from a couple of hours to overnight. When you cook it, it will almost taste like that oozy, fatty, a-butter-knife-will-cut-it prime meat.

Remember, we said *almost.*

"In marinating you not only build in the flavor but also make it more tender," says Lobel, who along with his brother has authored *Meat, All about Meat, How to Be Your Own Butcher* and *The Lobel Brothers Meat Cookbook.*

"The only thing you might have to add to the dressing is lots of garlic if that's what you like. That would definitely do the trick. And it would be quite good. Of course, you're still going to miss the flavor of a real prime piece of meat. It's a give-and-take situation."

If you want to be daring, you can mix up your own marinade. Make it a quarter acid and three-quarters oil, Lobel suggests. The acid softens the meat and the oil carries the flavors into the meat once the acid has softened it. For your acid you can use anything from wine to vinegar to lemon juice. Any cooking oil will do, although olive oil is preferred by some.

Be a Hamburger Helper

Hamburgers are as American as, well, apple pie. They're also just as fattening. A typical burger or slice of apple pie each packs more than 13 grams of fat.

We're not about to advise you to go burgerless on the Fourth of July—or any other time, for that matter, provided you're keeping your meat consumption within recommended guidelines. (Remember, two card decks a day.) But there are some simple steps you can take to significantly cut the fat in your burger.

Blot and drain. After browning ground beef, place it in a dish covered with a double-

Are You Game for New Meats?

Meat and potatoes is definitely a manly meal. And Broken Arrow Ranch general manager Perrin Wells doesn't suspect that men will ever replace their beef with rattlesnake.

They might try the bony morsel. They might boast about trying it. But eat it every day? Never.

"Everybody wants to say they've tried it. I've never seen anybody who lives on it," says Wells, whose Ingram, Texas, ranch sells deer, antelope, wild boar, rattlesnake and emu for human consumption.

But, unlike rattlesnake, some exotic fare—antelope and maybe ostrich—might not be considered so exotic at even the most finicky dinner tables of the future. Game meat and exotic birds have a chance to cut into the traditional beef and poultry markets simply because much of it tastes like beef and poultry. But it's much healthier. It all goes back to the home on the range. Because wild game have space to run around, most are significantly lower in fat and contain none of the hormones, large doses of antibiotics and other chemical injections that can be found in mass-produced farm animals.

So far, meat from game and exotic birds is mostly sold in restaurants. Some, however, is being sold in grocery stores near the ranches in states such as Texas and Colorado. And it can be ordered by mail or by phone. To order, get cooking tips or for general information on game meats, you can contact: Broken Arrow Ranch, P.O. Box 530, Ingram, TX 78025, 1-800-962-4263, or Colorado

thickness paper towel. Then stick another paper towel on top and blot up the grease. If you want to remove even more fat, dump the ground meat into a colander and rinse with

Mountain Game, 825 Denver Avenue, Fort Lupton, CO 80621, (303) 659-9219.

Here's a sampling of what might be considered a hearty meal sometime down the road.

• Ostrich. It's a red meat, but it has only about 2 grams of fat per 3.5-ounce portion, compared with 9.6 grams of fat in the same amount of broiled top loin. So far, ranches are primarily breeding these birds, says Bill Rowe, a sales representative at Colorado Mountain Game. And it's an expensive business. One pair of birds can run a farmer as much as $10,000, so the early ostrich steaks will be mucho expensive. Prices, however, are dropping, so keep your eyes open.

• Emu. It looks like a small ostrich, weighing in at 25 pounds when de-boned. The bird sells for between $6 and $10 a pound—about three times the price of steak. And that may be one big reason why people so far have only sampled the red-meat bird.

• Alligator. It's considered a seafood. And some say it tastes similar to halibut. Others say it tastes like a combination of chicken, rabbit and frog legs. It has about three grams of fat per 3.5-ounce portion. Usually the tail is the most tender. The tougher body meat is used for gumbo and stews.

• Antelope. It tastes like veal. The light-colored, fine-grained meat is about as lean as it gets, with only 2.7 grams of fat per 3.5 ounces. It is one of the most popular wild game selections.

• Rattlesnake. They bread it and deep-fry it. And it tastes, well, like rattlesnake.

"It looks like a rubbery catfish-colored meat. They're bony but not too meaty. It definitely has its own flavor, " says Wells.

---

can cut 50 percent of the fat from the beef.

Chill out. Once you've blotted and rinsed the meat, stick it in the refrigerator overnight. Whatever fat is left will harden. Then you can scrape it off the next day, says Nancy D. Berkoff of the Los Angeles Trade Technical College. Obviously, if you're the type of person who figures out what you're having for dinner a half-hour before you plan on eating it, this won't work for you.

Extend it. Remember Hamburger Helper? It will make your ground beef go a lot farther on a lot less fat. But the commercial product is also high in salt, so make your own hamburger helper. Mixing in bread crumbs, oatmeal, matzo meal, diced carrots and other vegetables will add bulk and cut down on the amount of meat you're eating.

Pay the price. Now that you know how to de-fat your ground beef, don't think you can buy the cheaper, higher-fat kind and make it healthy at home. You're wasting your money. The bulk in the cheaper beef will be from fat. Once you de-fat it, you'll have a lot less meat. It actually makes more sense to your wallet to purchase the more expensive, lower-fat meat, says Berkoff.

Order that burger well-done. Bacteria grows on the surface of beef, so grilling a steak on both sides will probably kill all of it regardless of how red it is on the inside. Hamburgers, though, are a different story. The surfaces of the ground beef that were exposed to air during the grinding process were spread throughout the burger when you made it, so you need to cook a burger until the center is gray.

---

hot, but not boiling, water. Squeeze out the excess water. The water will wash away fat and cholesterol while leaving the protein, iron, zinc and B_{12} behind. Using both of these methods

Deli

Make Your Sandwich a Cut above the Rest

Lunch just wouldn't feel like lunch without a killer sandwich. You know what we mean. One of those meat-packed, it-takes-two-hands, this-doesn't-fit-in-my-mouth sandwiches.

A killer it is. Sandwiches are made of things such as salami slices, which get 73 percent of their calories from fat, and provolone cheese, which gets about 68 percent of its calories from fat. And ham, which is 52 percent fat by calorie. And mayonnaise, which packs 11 grams of fat in just one tablespoon, getting 99 percent of its calories from fat.

You only need to examine the fat content of an Italian hoagie to get the picture. Even a somewhat puny one—four slices of salami, four slices of ham, four slices of provolone cheese, a couple of tablespoons of mayo and one hoagie roll—dumps 84.6 grams of fat and 1,376 calories into your system, which adds up to a whopping 55 percent of calories coming from fat.

Trimming the Fat

Used to be, just about anything that was called lunchmeat was bad for you. Hot dogs, pastrami, pepperoni. The rule was: If it tastes good, eat it.

But today, fat is public enemy number one, the Al Capone of the food world. And deli-meat makers have changed their artery-clogging ways. There are still horrifically fatty meats and cheeses out there, but there also are some lean choices that expand your sandwich menu beyond sliced turkey breast on whole-wheat bread.

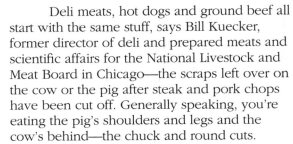

Deli meats, hot dogs and ground beef all start with the same stuff, says Bill Kuecker, former director of deli and prepared meats and scientific affairs for the National Livestock and Meat Board in Chicago—the scraps left over on the cow or the pig after steak and pork chops have been cut off. Generally speaking, you're eating the pig's shoulders and legs and the cow's behind—the chuck and round cuts.

Higher-fat deli meats usually start with scraps that are 70 percent lean says Kuecker. Lower-fat meats use 90 percent lean cuts.

By trimming fat and adding water and some nonmeat ingredients such as soy or other vegetables, the lower-fat meats can be transformed into relatively healthy eats.

Lean on Meat

You don't have to sacrifice taste to eat right. If you follow these suggestions, you can build a huge, it-takes-coordination-to-eat monstrosity of a sandwich that even Dagwood Bumstead would love. And you can save your heart for Blondie.

Go with the grain. Bread is your sandwich's foundation. Whole-grain breads will provide more fiber and minerals than white bread, says Neva Cochran, R.D., a private nutrition consultant and a spokesperson for the American Dietetic Association in Dallas. Don't be fooled by breads that look dark. Their dark color could be from molasses. She recommends you make sure the package says "whole grain."

Know the process. Processed meats such as bologna and salami are usually packed with fat and salt, but some traditionally high-fat stuff that now has no fat. Check the label to see how much fat you're getting for your calories, suggests Kuecker. By law, cold cuts labeled low-fat must have three grams or less per two-ounce serving.

Don't get whistled for piling on. Don't put a lot of meat or cheese on the sandwich, advises Cochran. Think of those items more like condiments that go with your vegetables. "There are a lot of options that are lean," she says. "It doesn't have to just be turkey or chicken. There's lean roast beef, lean ham, lower-fat cheese. Sometimes the amount of meat put on a sandwich is just as detrimental as the type. One thing you can do is put on less meat and more vegetables."

Veg out. The mark of any good sandwich is mouth-fitting ability. It should be small enough that you can get it in your mouth but wide enough that you can barely get it in your mouth. And the trick to making a bulky sandwich involves vegetables. Pile on leafy lettuce, tangy tomatoes, peppers, onions, cucumbers, sprouts—whatever occurs to you, says Cochran. Now, open wide.

Banish bacon. Bacon, lettuce and tomato sandwiches are the exception to rock singer Meat Loaf's bombastic ballad, "Two out of Three Ain't Bad." True, the lettuce and tomato are great, but the bacon makes this a less than healthy choice. From a fat and calorie standpoint, you'd be better off eating meat loaf. Instead of regular bacon, try turkey bacon or lean Canadian bacon, suggests Cochran.

Hold the mayo. Creamy dressings, mayonnaise and oil pack on fat and calories. Use mustard or look for low-fat varieties and use them sparingly, says Cochran.

Wrap it right. There's nothing worse than going to the fridge with a huge sandwich on your mind and discovering that the meat is sticky, slimy and, well, just gross. Lunchmeat generally lasts about four days after opening. To keep your meat fresh as long as possible, wrap it airtight in wax paper, says Stanley Lobel, a butcher and author of *All about Meat*.

Don't Ask, We'll Tell

It's the question no one who eats bologna wants to ask: What's in this stuff?

Bologna comes from the scraps left over after steaks and roasts have been chopped from the cow and pig. Up to 85 percent of it can come from such spare parts as hearts, tongues, livers and stomachs. By law, if the meat contains more than 40 percent of these spare parts, the package must say so and list which ones.

Now, just add some additives.

- **Salt.** Preserves the meat, flavors it and helps hold it together.
- **Nitrite.** Wards off botulism, serves as a powerful antioxidant, improves the flavor and gives the meat that nice pink color.
- **Ascorbic acid, erythorbic acid, sodium erythorbate, sodium ascorbate, citric acid, sodium citrate and sodium acid pyrophosphate.** They speed up the curing process and act as color stabilizers in the finished product.
- **Sugars.** Counteract the high salty flavor.
- **BHA (butylated hydroxyanisole), BHT (butylated hydroxytoluene) and propyl gallate.** Prevent rancidity.
- **Phosphates.** Improve the texture and help protect and stabilize the color and flavor of the finished product.
- **Potassium sorbate.** Prevents mold.
- **Extenders (cereal flour, nonfat dry milk, soy protein and sodium caseinate).** Lower the price because they make more with less. Also enhance the texture and flavor.
- **Spices.** Paprika, coriander, onion powder, monosodium glutamate, mace, ginger, cloves and garlic powder make it taste better.

Condiments

Spread Yourself Thin

Condiments are easy to forget. Sure, we remember to put them on our sandwiches. But we forget that we ate them. Not long ago, nutritionists at Washington State University in Pullman checked what college students really ate versus what they remembered eating. Half the time, the students forgot to mention their condiments.

Problem is, all those nonmemorable dabs here and there add fat and salt to your diet—and flab to your gut.

"One thing that really adds calories and fat to a sandwich is the kind of bread spread that you put on," says Neva Cochran of the American Dietetic Association. "So the alternative would be to use a lighter mayonnaise, or use mustard instead. Mustard has almost no fat."

Condiments are the things we put on our sandwiches to make them taste better. And mayo and the creamy dressings made from it are probably the biggest evils in the condiment world. One tablespoon of real mayonnaise packs almost 11 grams of fat—about 15 percent of the amount of fat a 170-pound guy should eat in a day. And for people concerned about their salt intake, there's soy sauce with as much as 3,300 milligrams of sodium per quarter-cup. You only need 2,400 milligrams a day.

You don't, however, have to give up flavoring your food and wetting your bread. Food should be enjoyed. To cut fat and salt, though, you should make some changes.

Change of Habit

There are plenty of other condiments that will give you

the illusions of salt and fat. Here are some suggestions

Don't pass mustard. It's low in salt and fat, and high in taste. Not a bad combination for something that's good for you. The only mustard to watch out for is the one combined with mayonnaise. These mustard-mayo combos have the same amount of fat as reduced-fat mayo. So they're better than real mayo but worse than regular mustard.

Catch up with ketchup. Though not as healthy as mustard, the tomato concentrate mixed with sugar, vinegar and some other flavorings isn't so bad for you, says James Kenney, R.D., Ph.D., a nutrition research specialist at the Pritikin Longevity Center in Santa Monica, California. Generally, you get more salt from ketchup because you use much more of it than mustard. And ketchup tends to keep bad company; we use it on french fries, hot dogs and hamburgers. So if you use it in moderation—a tablespoon or less—and put it on healthy foods, you'll do okay. You may also want to keep an eye out for those that have less sugar than leading brands or no salt added.

Substitute salsa. Dump it on your potato. Put it on everything. Unlike most condiments, salsa can actually be good for you, particularly if you use one that's low in sodium, says Dr. Kenney. Look for one that has less than 140 milligrams of sodium per serving. In addition to being packed with vegetables, salsa just might speed up your metabolism, provided you get the really, really hot stuff. And that will burn calories faster. But beware: If you get it too hot, chances are you'll be tempted to put out the hot pepper fire in your mouth with stuff you're trying to avoid—fatty foods, like milk, sour cream, ice cream or alcohol.

Be adventurous. Remember: We eat for pleasure,

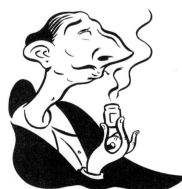

not just for survival. So don't fall into the rut of dumping mustard, ketchup or low-fat mayonnaise on your sandwiches. Anything hot and anything sweet will make a sandwich taste better. Experiment with hot pepper sauces, relishes and jellies. Try to use the sweeter stuff sparingly because it can pack some calories from sugar. "It takes experimenting with what tastes good to you and trying to cut back the amount. Slowly wean yourself back," says Robin Bagby, R.D., program development specialist for the College of Health and Human Development at Pennsylvania State University in University Park.

Use yogurt. Plain, unflavored yogurt can take on the taste of just about anything. Drain the liquid (whey) out of it through a cheesecloth, and use the leftover yogurt cheese as a substitute for cream cheese. Use it for sour cream. Use it for mayo. At first you'll notice the difference. But after a while, you'll get used to it. "You're not kidding anybody to say it's a substitute for cream cheese because it's not going to cook the same or set the same. But in some recipes it's an acceptable alternative," Bagby says.

Go from bad to Worcestershire. Many people avoid this condiment in the mistaken belief that it's high in salt. It only has 147 milligrams per tablespoon—making it a good alternative to using soy sauce, says Anita Hirsch, R.D., a nutritionist at the Rodale Food Center in Emmaus, Pennsylvania.

Be a bean counter. Really, this isn't as bad as it might sound. Drain some canned white beans and puree them in a blender with lemon juice, some garlic, some white wine, Worcestershire sauce and Dijon mustard. According to Susan

Massaron, food specialist and director of the cooking school at the Pritikin Longevity Center in Santa Monica, California, it makes a great, fiber-rich bread spread, as well as a dip.

Gotta Larva Livin' to Do

If you're bugged by the high fat content of most condiments, you might want to consider edible insects.

"Worms and insects are a traditional food for most people except for Europeans and us," says Gene DeFoliart, Ph.D., professor emeritus of entomology at the University of Wisconsin in Madison and founder and former editor of the *Food Insect Newsletter*, which has about 3,000 subscribers. "Right now there's much more interest than ever before in this," Dr. DeFoliart says.

Want to try making your own insect condiment? Come on. Be a real man. You can do it. Just go to any pet store and get a bunch of mealworms (a beetle larva used to make pet and zoo animal food). Then follow the advice of entomologist Ronald L. Taylor, Ph.D., in one of the few books written in the United States or Europe about insect eating, *Entertaining with Insects*.

Just mix up some cooked, minced mealworms with a package of low-fat cream cheese, some minced onions, low-fat milk, creamed horseradish, salt and pepper and bake it for 15 minutes at 350°F. Sprinkle with toasted, slivered almonds, and you have a great sandwich spread and dip.

Other edible insects in the United States include cicadas, crickets, bee pupa and wax worms. If you really want more information, you can subscribe to the *Food Insect Newsletter* by writing to Florence Dunkel at Montana State University's Department of Entomology, 324 Leon Johnson Hall, Bozeman, MT 59717.

Produce

Minding Your Peas and Cucumbers

It's a nightmare, that memory. Mom sticks a smushy, overcooked, sulphury-stinking plate of green balls on the table and bellows, "Eat." Yes, brussels sprouts—the name alone can cause a grown man to gag.

So imagine the stomach pains Ann Parker must have suffered when she started her new job. As public relations director of the Santa Cruz Beach Boardwalk, she had to promote the California amusement park's annual Brussels Sprouts Festival. She hated those tiny green balls. Hated them.

And here she had to convince people to come to a place that served brussels sprouts pizza, brussels sprouts ice cream, brussels sprouts cookies and brussels sprouts shish kebab for two days straight. Know what she did? She learned to like brussels sprouts.

Just goes to show, you can learn to like anything you set your mind to.

Fortunately, it doesn't have to be only brussels sprouts. But to boost your odds of preventing cancer and other assorted diseases, you should eat five to nine servings of fruits and vegetables a day, says Jerianne Heimendinger, R.D., Ph.D., former director of the National Cancer Institute's Five-a-Day-for-Better-Health! program based in Rockville, Maryland, and currently acting director of the Lifestyle Research Center at the AMC Cancer Research Center in Denver.

A serving is any of the following: three-quarters of a cup of 100 percent fruit juice, a medium-size piece of whole fruit, a half-cup of chopped veg-etables, a cup of salad greens, a quarter-cup of dried fruit or a half-cup of cut fruit or vegetables.

Help Yourself

At the buffet table of life the sign over the salad bar always reads, "All you can eat."

In general, produce contains only small amounts of those things doctors and nutritionists have been trying to get us to moderate: fat, calories and sodium. Produce has no cholesterol, and it is loaded with most of the stuff doctors say we need more of: fiber, vitamins A and C and antioxidants. It is also a good source of potassium, calcium and other minerals.

Fruits and vegetables contain hundreds of hard-to-pronounce and harder-to-spell cancer-fighting compounds known collectively as phytochemicals. About 35 percent of cancer deaths are thought to be related to diet. And in many studies, people who ate a lot of vegetables and fruits cut their risk of cancer in half compared to people who hardly touched the stuff.

While scientists have succeeded in identifying and isolating various phytochemicals from fruits and vegetables, cause-and-effect relationships have not been established in humans through clinical trials, says Clare Hasler, Ph.D., director of Functional Foods for Health, a joint program of the University of Illinois at Urbana-Champaign and Chicago.

Even so, doctors are pretty sure they know at least some of the phytochemicals that prevent cancer. Thing is, no one fruit or vegetable has all the phytochemicals. Tomatoes and watermelon have a particular kind of carotenoid that's different from the beta-carotene in carrots and sweet potatoes. Broccoli and brussels sprouts have anti-cancer compounds

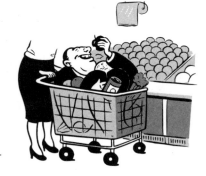

that are different from the cancer-fighting sulfurous compounds in garlic and onions. And citrus fruits have yet another compound called limonene.

Doctors believe those substances and a host of unknown others work in conjunction with one another to prevent many of the leading forms of cancer, so you can't just eat tons of the one fruit or one vegetable you like and say you got your five servings that day. You need a variety.

To get what is believed to be the essential phytochemicals in your diet, Dr. Hasler recommends eating something in these food categories everyday.

- Red fruits—tomatoes, watermelon, guavas, pink grapefruits
- Cruciferous vegetables—broccoli, cauliflower, brussels sprouts, cabbage
- Citrus—oranges, grapefruits and tangerines
- Tearjerkers—garlic and onions
- Orange vegetables—carrots, pumpkins, sweet potatoes

In addition to preventing cancer, eating fruits and vegetables also helps prevent stroke, heart disease and age-related blindness. Athletes should eat a lot of fruits and vegetables because their high water content replaces fluids and some electrolytes lost in perspiration.

If you're not that crazy about fruits and vegetables, you'll want to concentrate on those that produce the most nutritional bang for your buck with each serving. Here's a breakdown of some produce powerhouses recommended by the National Cancer Institute's Five-a-Day-for-Better-Health! program.

- Provides 50 percent of the recommended Daily Value for Vitamin A—apricots, can-

taloupes, bok choy, carrots, chile peppers, spinach, winter squash and sweet potatoes.

- Provides 50 percent of the recommended Daily Value for Vitamin C—broccoli, brussels sprouts, cauliflower, chili peppers, green

The Forbidden Fruit

Nutritionally, we know apples are good for us. Basically, the fiber-rich fruits help us stay regular guys.

But for centuries we've looked to apples to provide us with other benefits. Here are just a few.

- **To win races.** In Greek mythology the huntress Atalanta offered to marry any chap who could beat her in a race. The losers—and there were many—lost their lives. She speared them. But that didn't deter her suitors, one of whom was Milanion. Not relishing the idea of being speared to death, Milanion tricked her into losing. He dropped three golden apples as he raced. Atalanta stopped to pick them up and lost.

- **To make body parts.** We all know about how Eve fed Adam that apple. But what a lot of us don't know is exactly what happened once Adam ate it. Yeah, yeah. They got their eviction notice from Paradise. Eve was cursed with painful childbirth. But some people believe yet another thing happened that fateful day: Adam got a new body part. He never could manage to swallow that apple. It got stuck in his throat, and the Adam's apple was created.

- **To tell the future.** So you've been seeing this woman for a while. It's a promising relationship. You like her. Your friends like her. Heck, your dog likes her. But, well, you're still a little wary about tying the knot. What to do? Cut an apple in half. An even number of seeds means marriage is the way to go. But if you cut open a seed while slicing the apple, it means there's trouble in paradise.

peppers, grapefruits, kiwis, oranges, cantaloupes, papayas and strawberries.
- Provides four or more grams of fiber—figs, pears, prunes, dried peas and beans. (Most fruits and vegetables have between one and three grams.)

Learning to Like It

Okay, you're convinced. You *should* eat more vegetables. But you've known that for years. The problem is that you still don't *want* to eat them.

Most of us have no problem eating vitamin-vacant iceberg lettuce, but cruciferous vegetables, like bok choy, broccoli, brussels sprouts, cabbage and cauliflower, present a greater challenge. Some guys hate just about every vegetable imaginable except lettuce and carrots.

What makes one guy a vegetable lover and another a vegetable hater?

It might all come down to another hard-to-pronounce and harder-to-spell compound called 6-n-propyl-thiouracil. It seems people who are really sensitive to that are also pretty sensitive to both bitter and sweet tastes, says Ann Ferris, R.D., Ph.D., professor and head of the Department of Nutritional Sciences at the University of Connecticut in Storrs.

Researchers assume that there is a link between tasting that compound and dislike of bitter-tasting foods, but a link has never been definitely shown. And women seem to be more sensitive to 6-n-propyl-thiouracil than men, Dr. Ferris says.

That doesn't mean you're a girly man if the thought of stomaching brussels sprouts or

Sprouting Your Wings

Now we're not going to force you to eat brussels sprouts. We're not your mother. But we're going to let you in on a few secrets that might help you make those little green balls go down easier. Here's the reasoning: If you can learn to like brussels sprouts, you can learn to like anything.

First, you should know that until the mid-1960s, sprouts were handpicked. Then came a revolution. By crossbreeding different kinds of sprouts, scientists created a variety that could be machine harvested.

"A lot of the characteristics were fine for farming, but the one characteristic that they didn't pay a lot of attention to was taste," says Steve Bontadelli, a brussels sprouts grower in Santa Cruz, California, the sprouts capital of the United States. "So they were real bitter, and that's what a lot of people in our generation were raised on. They never tried them again."

Today, however, brussels sprouts science has far surpassed what it was in the 1960s. Today's hybrids are better tasting and milder. Some are even, shall we go so far as to say, sweet.

There's one bad characteristic that has not been bred out of today's sprouts. They still stink. Not to worry.

cooked celery makes you queasy. It just means researchers are not quite sure why so many of us hate vegetables so much.

Possibly, vegetable hating is partly socialization, Dr. Ferris says.

"When you're a child, there's an assumption that you're not going to like brussels sprouts. There's an assumption that nobody's going to like brussels sprouts," she says. "A lot of it is that we're socialized as children not to like them."

That's why some doctors feel you can

You can do something about that smell. Cook them with a few celery stalks. That goes for any stinky vegetable.

Also, you want to flavor them. Garlic is a great complement. Or if you have a roast in the oven, toss in some frozen sprouts during the last half-hour to let them soak up the meat juices.

Some other sprout strategies:

Avoid the middle, man. **Buy sprouts either in the late season (December to January) or the early season (July to September). Those varieties are milder than ones grown during other times of the year.**

Baby them. **Buy younger, smaller sprouts. They're milder.**

Let X mark the spot. **When preparing them, cut an X in the butt to make them cook evenly. And whatever you do—and this goes for all vegetables—don't overcook them. Smushy brussels sprouts rank as one of the ultimate gross-out foods. "That's another thing our moms used to do a lot, cook the heck out of them. Then there's this yucky, mushy thing you eat," says Bontadelli. "They are much better al dente. You can put a fork in them, but you don't want them to mush out."**

make yourself like or at least tolerate your most-despised vegetable by simply eating it a lot.

And that's how Ann Parker learned to like brussels sprouts. As a part of the Santa Cruz Brussels Sprouts Festival, she tried them in pizza. She had them stir-fried. She had them spun into saltwater taffy.

"The big surprise was, I think I only had two dishes I didn't like during the five years I promoted it," Parker says. "It's like any food. You have to prepare it correctly. People would come to the festival thinking they hated them,

then they would taste some of the recipes and they would change their minds."

Produce More

If you want to increase your produce consumption, you have to think produce. All the time.

"Try and incorporate it into every meal," Dr. Hasler says. "Just really try to make it a part of your diet. It's a major behavior and dietary change. If you're eating three meals a day and two or three snacks, you should have your five servings right there."

Meal by meal, here are some easy ways to get more produce into your diet.

Breakfast

- Drink six ounces of orange juice.
- Put a half-cup of fruit (sliced bananas, strawberries, blueberries) on your cereal or pancakes.
- Eat a bowl of fruit.

Snacks

- Instead of coffee or a soda, have six ounces of 100 percent fruit juice such as pineapple, grapefruit or orange. Drinking a blend of different fruits and vegetables is great because it provides more than one type of phytochemical.
- Try nonfat fruit bars, whole fruit (apples, bananas) or cut vegetables for snacks instead of candy.

Lunch

- Have a salad. To cut down on preparation time, make it at the grocery store salad bar or buy presliced, bagged lettuce and vegetables. A large salad with two cups of leafy greens can count for two or more servings. Try to mix in lots of different-colored vegetables. Besides making your salad prettier, it increases the number of phytochemicals.

- Eat vegetables such as carrots or celery sticks on the side, or eat a piece of fruit.
- Add lettuce, tomato, sprouts and other vegetables to your sandwiches.

Dinner

- Make vegetables a part of the main dish. Stir-fry chicken with broccoli or snow peas.
- Have a salad.
- Garnish the main dish with sliced fruit.

Dessert

- Stick fruit on top of cake or ice cream.

Making Time

Probably the biggest reason you don't eat enough produce is the time factor. You may have time to buy a head of broccoli. Then it sits in the fridge. Sits in the fridge. Sits in the fridge. Then you notice a gooey, slimy growth. Time to chuck it.

Don't be so traditional. There are lots of ways to get produce into your diet.

Shake it. Instead of letting the stuff sit in the fridge, shove it in the blender and make a shake out of it. One example is fresh strawberries with orange juice. Or make grapefruit juice ice cubes and stick them in pineapple juice.

Bag it. Buy prepackaged, already-sliced items to snack on at home. These can include canned pears, sliced watermelon and baby carrots. Make sure canned fruits are packed in 100 percent fruit juice. You may think you're getting fewer vitamins when someone else does the cutting. Not true. Research shows that bagged vegetables don't breathe as much as unbagged vegetables. That

means they use up fewer nutrients.

Cut it. Wash and cut up vegetables such as carrots, celery and zucchini for easy access. Wrap them in plastic or keep them in water to keep them fresh.

Stash it. Store items where you'll find them, such as your briefcase, your car or your desk.

Cool it. Keep small bottles or cans of 100 percent fruit juice in the fridge. That way you can grab one to drink on the way to work.

Grab it. Have a piece of fruit such as a banana or apple handy. Bring easy-to-eat fruits and vegetables to eat in the car. Top choices include apples, bananas, carrots, grapes and pears. Keep dried fruits—prunes, raisins, peaches, figs—in the glove compartment.

Freeze it. Put bagged vegetables you're not going to eat soon in the freezer to make them last.

Keeping It Fresh

If no self-respecting man would stop to ask for directions to some place he really wants to go, then he's sure as hell not going to ask some supermarket produce manager for directions on how to store fruits and vegetables. We understand that. So to make your life simpler, Kathy Means, vice-president of membership and public affairs for the Produce Marketing Association in Newark, Delaware, has provided a list of handling tips for 20 commonly used fruits and vegetables. All of these are available year-round.

- Bananas. Store them at room temperature to ripen. Refrigerate ripe (yellow with black specks) bananas. It will turn the skins black, but the insides will be fine. They will keep a few days, depending on the stage of ripeness.
- Apples. Either store them at room temperature or in the fridge. They will keep for weeks if refrigerated.
- Oranges. Their peak season is October

through May. You can store them at room temperature if you plan to eat them within two weeks. Otherwise, store in the refrigerator. They'll keep for weeks there. To get juicier oranges, pick out those that seem heavy for their size.

- Cantaloupes. Store ripe ones in the fridge, where they will last a few days. You cannot judge ripeness by thumping. Ripe ones have a cantaloupe smell and can be pressed at the blossom end.

- Grapes. Store them in a plastic bag in the fridge. They'll keep there for a few days. Wash them before serving, not before storing.

- Avocados. Store ripe ones in the warmest part of the refrigerator for up to three days. You can ripen them at home by putting them in a loosely closed paperbag at room temperature. Keep checking them, because there is a fine line between ripeness and over-ripeness. When they yield to gentle pressure, they're ready to eat. You can get them to ripen faster by sticking a ripe banana or tomato in the bag. The fruit will give off a natural gas that will heat up the bag and help the avocado ripen.

- Lemons. You can store them at room temperature for a few days or, for longer storage, keep whole lemons in the fridge up to a month. Before using, stick the fruit in the microwave for ten seconds, then roll it on a countertop before squeezing to release more juice.

- Strawberries. Their peak season is April through August. Store them unwashed in the refrigerator. They'll keep for a few days. Wash before eating.

- Peaches. Their peak season is April through October. Ripen them at room temperature and refrigerate them when ripe. They'll keep for a few days in the refrigerator. Buy firm but slightly soft peaches with yellow between the red

parts. Ripe ones smell peachy.

- Grapefruit. Their peak season is January through June. You can store them a few days at room temperature and a week or more in the refrigerator. Choose heavy fruit.

- Potatoes. Store them in a cool, dry, dark place for up to two months. Refrigeration will alter the taste.

- Head lettuce. To make it last longer, core it by slamming it against something (some guys use the wall, others the counter) and then ripping off the stem. Rinse, drain and stick it in a tightly closed bag or container in the crisper section of the refrigerator. Whole lettuce will last about a week.

- Tomatoes. Store at room temperature until ripe, then eat immediately. Once a tomato is sliced, it should be refrigerated or it will quickly go bad. But be fore-warned: Tomatoes lose their taste in the fridge.

- Onions. Store in a cool, dry, dark place with good air circulation in a loosely woven bag, basket or crate. They'll keep for weeks. Refrigerate cut onions in a covered container.

- Carrots. Remove the green tops and store unwashed in a plastic bag in the refriger-ator. They store well for two weeks.

- Broccoli. Put it unwashed in a plastic bag in the crisper. It will last up to three days.

- Cucumbers. Refrigerate, either cut or whole, in a plastic bag. An unpeeled cu-cumber will last for a week.

- Bell peppers. Store in a plastic bag in the fridge for up to five days.

- Cauliflower. Store it unwashed in a plastic bag in the crisper. It can keep for a week, but eat it as soon as possible to avoid a strong taste and smell.

- Mushrooms. Refrigerate them in a paper bag. They will last up to two days. Wash them before eating, not storing.

Dairy

Moo-ve toward Better Health

The cow looks like a slacker. It stands around. Eats some grass. Chews. Stares into space. Chews. Takes a nap. Chews. Stares into space. Chews.

But its production abilities are awesome. Because of its four-compartment stomach, the cow can eat vitamin-packed, non-human-digestible grass, spit it up, chew on it, choke it back down and eventually make milk we can drink. That milk is turned into an array of foods, from cheese to butter to yogurt.

Though eggs are not technically a dairy food—they're not made from milk—we'll be talking about them later in this chapter because you usually find them next to the milk cartons in the grocery store.

It Does a Body Good

Though buffalo and goats supply milk and related products for various parts of the world, the cow has the U.S. market cornered.

How does it get from farm to you? The thin, white liquid is pumped from the cow, cooled, processed, analyzed for bacterial count, heated to destroy bacteria, yeast and molds (this is called pasteurizing) and then cooled again.

Though not required by law, most milk is also homogenized by forcing the liquid through very small pressurized tubes that break up the fat and disperse it evenly. If milk was not homogenized, cream would rise to the top. Low-fat and skim milk are not always homogenized, however,

because much of the cream has been removed.

Packed with more than 40 nutrients, milk products provide a huge amount of essential vitamins and protein, including 75 percent of the calcium in the average American diet.

Calcium is what makes milk such a great food. That and the fact that you can guzzle it straight out of the carton. Three cups of milk, three cups of yogurt or three to five ounces of cheese will cover your Daily Value of calcium. That means strong bones and teeth. Adequate calcium intake also may help prevent colon cancer and high blood pressure.

If you don't like milk, though, don't feel like you have to drink it. Broccoli, kale, turnip greens, seeds and nuts are also considered good sources for calcium, but keep in mind that you'll have to eat a lot of them. You'll need 2½ cups of broccoli, 6 cups of pinto beans or 30 cups of soy milk in order to get the same amount of calcium that you would from an eight-ounce glass of milk.

Obviously, milk is the easier alternative. To get the most from your milk, you'll want to keep it cold and in the dark. Strong sunlight and fluorescent light will destroy vitamins. And milk should be stored below 44°F to prevent bacteria growth.

Skim the Fat

The problem with milk and milk products is that many are high in fat. Whole milk gets nearly 50 percent of its calories from fat, and Cheddar cheese packs a whopping 74 percent of its calories from fat.

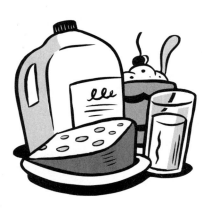

Fortunately, if you're concerned about fat, you don't have to give up milk products. You just need to give up the ones high in fat. One of the simplest ways to do that is to switch to skim or low-fat milk and milk products. Researchers have found that simply switching from whole milk to skim could reduce cholesterol levels by 7 percent.

What's the difference between low-fat and skim? Milk is labeled low-fat if it's less than 2 percent fat by weight. Sounds pretty good, doesn't it? It's not. Two percent milk still gets 30 percent of its calories from fat. One percent milk gets 20 percent of its calories from fat.

Skim milk has as much fat removed as is technologically possible. Skim milk gets 6 percent of its calories from fat, and all of the good stuff is left in.

"When the fat changes, nothing else does," says Pennsylvania State University's Robin Bagby. "Skim milk is still a good source of protein. That hasn't changed. It's a good source of calcium. That hasn't changed. It's only less fat."

Switching to skim milk may be more palatable if you do it in small steps. If you're used to drinking whole milk, first try 2 percent. Then go down to 1 percent and work your way down to skim. Try different brands of skim. You might find one brand more palatable than another, says Bagby.

Margarine versus Butter

First they told you butter is loaded with artery-clogging saturated fat. So you switched to margarine. Then they said margarine is loaded with artery-clogging trans-fatty acids. So you decided you may as well eat whatever you damn well please because the doctors can't make up their minds.

But the butter versus margarine debate really isn't all that complicated. The bottom line is this: They're both bad for you.

There's no disagreement over the evils of butter's saturated fat. It clogs your arteries. The consensus of the health world is to limit saturated fat to no more than 10 percent of your daily calories.

Margarine's trans-fatty acids are bad, too.

Studies have shown that both saturated fat and trans-fats increase your risk of coronary heart disease because they lower HDL, the good cholesterol, and raise LDL, the bad cholesterol. The problem is that nutritionists can't tell you to keep your intake to a particular amount because you have no way to gauge how much of the stuff you're eating. Unlike saturated fat, trans-fats aren't listed on food labels. If you see partially hydrogenated vegetable oil on the list of ingredients, you know the food has trans-fatty acids lurking inside. But you have no way of knowing how much.

What's a health-conscious guy to do?

Jump in the tub. If you have to choose, margarine with low trans-fats is likely to be the healthier alternative, says Harvard University's Dr. Walter C. Willett. In a tablespoon serving, margarine has two grams of saturated fat compared to butter's seven, and the margarine has no cholesterol. Go for the tub versions or liquid "squeeze" versions of low-fat or nonfat margarines. The softer the margarine, the less trans-fatty acids. Here's a list of some low saturated fat and low trans-fatty acid products that the folks at the Center for Science in the Public Interest have given their stamp of approval to: Fleischmann's Lower Fat Margarine, Promise Ultra, Weight Watchers Extra Light Spread, Parkay Light and Kraft Touch of Butter Spread.

Spread out. When cooking or baking, try to use oil instead of butter or margarine. For spreads, think of other things to smear on top: jam, honey, hot peppers, relish. "It's experimenting with what tastes good to you and trying to cut back and slowly weaning yourself back," says Bagby. "It's small steps over time."

Cut your hydrogenated fat. Hydrogenated fat is the main source of trans-fats, so cutting down on your intake of products that list hydrogenated or partially hydrogenated fat high on their list of ingredients should help reduce your trans-fat intake as well, says Dr. Willett.

Say Cheese

According to legend, cheese was discovered by accident. Several thousand years ago a guy stuck some milk in a sheep's stomach pouch and set out on a day-long journey. The heat and the stomach enzymes turned the milk into a snowy white cheese curd and a liquid called whey.

Sounds kind of unappetizing doesn't it? But we know the next time you see some Swiss cubes on a party tray, the memory of that story won't keep you from stuffing cube after cube into your mouth. Men like cheese. With most cheeses averaging 66 percent of their calories from fat, cheese is one of the most common fat boosters in our diet. Just one small 1½-inch cube of hard cheese takes care of a third of our day's maximum intake of saturated fat.

Good thing food scientists have figured out how to de-fat cheese by adding more milk protein and taking away milk's cream. But if you're used to eating regular cheese, don't expect these low-fat or nonfat versions to meet your taste standards, even though these versions are improving. To get the most out of them, substitute part of the regular cheese you're putting in a casserole, pasta salad or on a pizza with a nonfat or low-fat version, suggests Rodale's Anita Hirsch. That way, you'll still get the flavor of the regular cheese but with less of the fat. Another good reason to blend a regular cheese with its nonfat counterpart in a hot dish is that some of the nonfat cheeses don't melt very well. Some nonfat and low-fat cheeses that taste good, according to Hirsch, include Kraft ⅓ Less Fat Cheddar Singles Pasteurized Process Cheese Product, Borden Fat Free Process Cheese Product, Borden Lite Line Low Fat Sharp and Kraft Philadelphia Brand Light Cream Cheese.

Some other ways to de-fat your cheese.

Stay light, eat white. White cheeses such as mozzarella, Swiss, ricotta and Parmesan are generally lower in fat than yellow cheeses such as Cheddar and American because they are often made with low-fat milk instead of whole. Be aware, though, that food coloring can be used to make higher-fat cheeses white, so if you buy white American or white Cheddar cheese, you'll get just as much fat as you would in the yellow versions. In general, white cheeses also are good choices to buy in the low-fat variety. You won't miss the taste as much because white cheeses tend to have a milder flavor than yellow cheeses, says Gregory D. Miller, Ph.D., vice-president of nutrition research and technology transfer for the National Dairy Council in Rosemont, Illinois.

Make it old and hard. If you're going to eat the real heart-clogging stuff, then at least do your teeth some good. Have it for dessert. A few studies indicate that hard, aged cheeses such as Monterey Jack and Cheddar may reduce cavity-causing bacteria.

Melt it and hide it. Nonfat cheese tends to look like plastic when melted. So if you hide it in a casserole, you won't notice it as much.

Yogurt: The Wonder Dairy Food

It might reduce colon cancer. It might boost immunity. It might aid digestion. A cup a day just might make you live to be 100.

Thing is, these are all mights.

"There's some interesting data with the lactic acid bacteria that suggests it can change the bacteria in the colon. And it's certainly exciting data. I don't think it's proven. It's somewhat speculative, but it is consistent," says Dennis A. Savaiano, Ph.D., professor and dean of the School of Consumer and Family Sciences at Purdue University in West Lafayette, Indiana. "I think we're in the same stage with yogurt and immunity. The data looks promising, but this is a hard issue to prove."

Even with all the magical, life-enhancing qualities aside, yogurt is a nutritional powerhouse. A cup provides 300 to 450 milligrams of calcium, more than milk. It also supplies more B vitamins, phosphorus and potassium than milk. And a cup of low-fat yogurt gives you a fifth of your recommended daily protein intake.

Plain, nonfat yogurt can be used as a substitute for just about any fat-laden condiment, but some yogurts are better than others. Here's how to pick the best.

Get cultured. If your package of yogurt includes the statement "meets the National Yogurt Association criteria for live and active culture yogurt," it means the yogurt has at least ten million cultures per gram. And doctors think the bacteria give yogurt its health-promoting qualities. An easy way to be sure your yogurt contains significant amounts of these cultures is to look for the National Yogurt Association "LAC" seal on yogurt containers, says Timothy Morck, Ph.D., director of nutrition, regulatory and consumer affairs for the Dannon Company in Tarrytown, New York.

Zap the fat. Yogurt can get almost half of its calories from fat. Read the labels and choose the low-fat and nonfat varieties.

Consider the calcium. If you're lactose intolerant, you may consider using yogurt as your primary dairy product because the cultures aid in digestion. Just make sure to choose yogurt that supplies 20 to 40 percent of your Daily Value for calcium in an eight-ounce serving, says Dr. Morck.

Check the date. As yogurts with live cultures age, they continue to produce lactic acid, which causes them to have more of a "bite" or tart taste. You won't get sick eating them, but you may not like the way they taste, especially if you prefer a mild, sweet flavor, Dr. Morck says. Unless you or the supplier had the yogurt sitting in the hot sun, it will last at least until the date on the cup. That date is generally the last day the product should be sold in stores, he says, but you can feel confident eating most yogurts up to a week after the date expires. If you are concerned about eating it after the date

has expired, call the manufacturer's phone number, located on the product's container.

Keep the whey. When you open yogurt and there's some runny liquid floating on top, don't pour it out. It's whey. It contains protein and calcium. Stir it in, says Dr. Morck.

Lighten Your Yolk

For a while, eggs were portrayed as the ultimate evil in the food world. We're not going to tell you to start making omelets every morning. But we are going to remove some of the stigma.

The reason eggs got such a bad rap is because of the high amount of cholesterol they pack. Two eggs will put you well over your recommended Daily Value. But it seems we don't have to worry as much about dietary cholesterol as we once thought.

Still, no one's going to tell you to eat more than four eggs a week.

"When you have two eggs for breakfast, that's 400 milligrams of cholesterol that you've received at breakfast alone. Even if you go to a strict no-cholesterol diet for the rest of the day, you've already taken in more than the recommended amount, which is 300 milligrams. So a person who eats two eggs for breakfast plus bacon, which has cholesterol, and then goes on to eat regular meals will end up with probably 500, maybe 600 or 700, milligrams of cholesterol," says the USDA's Dr. Gary J. Nelson. "Even though cholesterol is less critical in raising your blood cholesterol level than dietary saturated fat, when you get up into 700 or 800 milligrams per day, it does have a significant effect."

Point is, you don't have to feel guilty every time you eat an egg. Just keep them to less than four times a week and don't cook them in butter.

You can cut some of the cholesterol from your omelet by not putting in as many yolks. According to Dr. Nelson, if you don't want to pick out the yolk yourself, buy egg substitutes.

Beer and Wine

The Power of Positive Drinking

Stupid machismo trick number 365: Strong arms hoist the body into a handstand on top of the keg. Lips suck ice cold beer from the tap as buddies chant the number of seconds tap and mouth stay intact.

The feat may garner lots of woofing noises and high fives among college crowds who think *Animal House* was a documentary, but real men don't drink like that.

"That whole idea of guzzling beer is really not what we're promoting," says Stephen Hindy, founder and president of Brooklyn Brewery, a New York City microbrewery. "Our idea is drink less but drink something better. Drink something interesting."

Beer—like a fine wine or single malt Scotch—should be smelled. It should be admired. And it should be savored, Hindy says. "If you learn to drink intelligently, you may do wonders for your health," says Arthur Klatsky, M.D., senior consultant in cardiology at Kaiser Permanente Medical Center in Oakland, California.

nondrinkers. Drinking raises the HDL—often called the "good" cholesterol—that scoops away the artery-clogging "bad" cholesterol known as LDL, says Dr. Klatsky. It also may hamper clot formation in the arteries by making blood less sticky, he says.

But Dr. Klatsky and other physicians won't tell you to take two beers and call in the morning. Some people can't stop at two drinks, Dr. Klatsky says. Once you have six or more a day, you have a higher rate of dying from coronary heart disease than teetotalers or moderate drinkers. You're also at risk for a number of other diseases, including cirrhosis of the liver.

If you already drink an average of two a day—whether that's 24 ounces of beer, 10 ounces of wine or 1¼ ounces of an 80-proof stiff one—there's no reason to stop, Dr. Klatsky says. Just remember that you can't save up your daily drinks and then go wild on a Friday night. It doesn't work that way, Klatsky says.

What's the optimal anti-heart-disease drink? There's some evidence that red wine has some components that lower cholesterol more effectively than other drinks. But ninety percent of wine's cholesterol-lowering effect comes from its alcohol content, so whether you drink wine, beer or whiskey, your risk of coronary heart disease will still be reduced, Klatsky says.

Drink for the Health of It

In countless bars over many generations, patrons have cheerily toasted, "To your health," before raising their glasses to their lips. Turns out they were right all along— provided you're only raising a glass or two. Studies show moderate drinkers—people who have one to two drinks a day— are less likely to die from coronary heart disease than

Appreciating the Finer Things

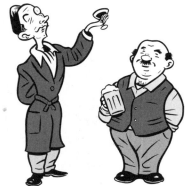

In the thousands of years that man has quaffed beer and wine, he has learned at least a thing or two about the fine art of drinking. Here are just a few.

Storage. Both beer and wine should be kept in a dark, cool place. Corked beverages should be stored on the side to keep the cork wet. If the cork dries out, it will shrink, allowing oxygen to get in the bottle, and you'll get stale wine. Also, light will ruin most aged wines and give beer a skunky taste. That's why wine and beer bottles are colored—to keep the light out.

How long? Some beers are dated. For those without expiration dates, plan to drink them within four months, because the flavor will deteriorate after that, says Hindy. Granted, for most guys this isn't a great concern. You can find out when your wine should be opened by using a vintage chart. You can get one for $5.00 (postage included) from the American Wine Society, 3006 Latta Road, Rochester, NY 14612. The 12-page booklet also includes information on wine storage and serving.

Serving. Both beer and wine pretty much follow the same rule. The lighter the color, the colder it should be. Clear beers and clear wines go from the fridge to the glass. "Don't keep white wines ice cold—you won't be able to enjoy their flavor," says Angel E. Nardone, director of the American Wine Society in Rochester, New York. "About 15 minutes before serving, put the wine in the refrigerator. By the time you're ready to pour, the wine will be chilled to the right temperature."

Red wine and dark beer, however, should be cool, not cold. Red wine tastes best when served at about 56°F. "Even full-bodied whites, like Chardonnays, should be served cool—probably about the same temperature as in your basement," says Nardone. "That's why wines are kept in cellars, it preserves their aroma and taste qualities."

Likewise, you can't taste the unique blend of hops (the bitter stuff) and malts (the sweet stuff) of a dark beer when it's cold. "The old American cold beer fixation I think has a lot to do with the lack of flavor in most mainstream American beers," Hindy says. "Microbrewers want you to taste the malt character

What's in It?

Following are the alcohol and caloric content of a 12-ounce serving of some popular beers.

Brand	Calories	% Alcohol (By Volume)
Busch	153	4.8
Busch Light	117	3.9
Bud Dry	130	4.8
Bud Light	110	4.2
Budweiser	142	4.8
Coors Light	103	4.2
Coors Premium	141	4.7
Guinness Extra Stout	181	5.8
Killian's	172	5.4
Miller Genuine Draft	147	4.7
Miller Genuine Draft Light	98	4.2
Pete's Wicked Ale	170	5.0
Pilsner Urquell	150	5.5
Samuel Adams Boston Lager	160	4.9
Schmidt's	142	4.6

and the hop character in their beers. If it's ice cold, a lot of the complexity in the beer gets masked."

Pouring. It's a question that can keep a beer drinking group arguing for hours: Should the beer be poured down the side or straight into the glass? The answer: It depends. Some beers are carbonated out the wazoo. "If you would pour them in the bottom of the glass, you would have them in your lap. They're very explosive beers," Hindy says.

But most beers should be poured directly into the bottom of the glass. That allows a head to form, which, despite popular American belief, is a good thing. All good beers should have a head at least the width of two fingers, Hindy says. Having a good head allows the carbon dioxide to escape from the beer. That means less burping, and it also makes the beer perfectly sniffable.

Other Beverages

Whet Your Appetite for Good Health

You just don't see parched lizards desperately in search of an oasis. Even if the desert sand stretched out to the horizon, there would be little need for reptilian concern. Various glands and excretions would keep the lizard's body running despite its desiccated state.

No wonder desiccated rock star Jim Morrison wanted to be the Lizard King. We mere humans don't have such amazing abilities. We need a lot of water. The liquid carries nutrients from our food throughout our bodies, takes waste through the intestines, lubricates our joints, organs and other body parts and oozes through our pores as sweat to keep our body temperature at about 98°F. It's so important, about 60 percent of our bodies are comprised of water.

We get some of our water from food; watermelon is 92 percent water, lettuce 96 percent. Even so, to keep all those functions running smoothly, nonactive adults should drink a half-ounce of water per pound of body weight per day. That means a 160-pound person should down ten eight-ounce glasses. Active people should drink even more, about two-thirds of an ounce for each pound.

Make Juice Your Main Squeeze

Drinking fruit or vegetable juices is a great way to satisfy two dietary needs. It helps quench your body's thirst for water. And if you drink the

right kind, you can get in some of the fruit and vegetable servings so many of us are lacking. Many juices are great sources of vitamin C, providing anywhere from 10 to 100 percent of the Daily Value in each eight-ounce serving. Some are also good sources of calcium and beta-carotene. The only difference between juice and the real fruit or vegetable is that most juices lack the fiber. And you'll recall that fiber helps protect men from colon cancer and high cholesterol. So don't think you can get all of your fruits and vegetables out of a glass.

Still, there are several reasons why it's a good idea to squeeze juice into your daily diet. All citrus juices have vitamin C, some as much as twice the Daily Value in an eight-ounce glass. Beta-carotene—an antioxidant that is believed to help guard against cancer and boost immunity—can be found in most red- or orange-colored juices. Potassium can be found in nearly all juices, especially carrot, prune, tomato and orange. Prune juice is the only one high in iron. One cup provides 17 percent of the Daily Value. Surprisingly, fortified orange juice has as much calcium as milk.

The problem is that some juice drinks can be deceiving.

Here's how to make sure that you're getting the real deal.

Read the label. Any juice that claims to be 100 percent juice really is. Anything that says it's 10 percent juice really is. Remember, it's a glass of 100 percent juice that counts as one produce serving. The choice is yours: Drink 8 ounces of real fruit juice or 80 ounces of a 10 percent juice drink, beverage, punch or blend. The biggest difference is all the empty calories you'll pile on to get the same health benefit.

Inspect the ingredients. They are listed in order of decreasing quantity. So the first ingredient is always the most prevalent in the drink.

Look for juices that have juice and not water listed first. "Even if it's not 100 percent juice, at least it has more juice than water," says Neva Cochran of the American Dietetic Association.

Keep a lid on it. Over time, oxygen and light can rob any juice of its vitamins, Cochran says. Make sure to keep lids tightly closed. And check dates. Orange juice may start to lose its flavor once it has lost vitamins. So chances are—regardless of whether it's from concentrate or fresh squeezed—it will give you 100 percent of your vitamin C Daily Value if it tastes like orange juice and if you use it before the date stamped on the container. Orange juice usually lasts two to four weeks in a home fridge before there's a serious loss of vitamin C and taste.

Watch What You Drink

If you have a cup of coffee with breakfast, a soda with lunch and a bottle of beer with dinner, how much of your daily water requirement have you satisfied? Zero. Zilch. Nada. That's because caffeinated and alcoholic beverages are diuretics—they actually rob your body of water.

Not only do they not count, it's probably a good idea to drink even more water if you consume such beverages.

Regular, nondiet soda also packs another minus—lots of empty calories. Unless you have a weight problem, however, you probably don't need to give it up.

Here are some ways to make your diet more fluid.

Take a break. Instead of coffee, take water breaks, recommends Cochran. Try to drink water every 30 to 45 minutes.

Fuel up before meals. You can take the edge off your appetite by downing a glass of

Water, Water Everywhere

When the Food and Drug Administration inspected bottled waters, they discovered that about 25 percent of them were nothing more than regular municipal water in a bottle.

So, like the good government agency they are, they came up with some regulations. Here's a guide to reading bottled water labels.

- **Mineral water.** It was tapped at a borehole or spring that came from a geologically and physically protected underground water source.
- **Spring water.** It came from underground, flowed naturally to the surface and was collected at the spring itself or through a borehole next to the spring.
- **Distilled.** The water was vaporized and then condensed to get rid of dissolved minerals. Of all the bottled waters, distilled is one of the safest to drink.
- **Purified.** The water has been distilled, deionized (passed through resins that remove most of the dissolved minerals), put through reverse osmosis (membrane filters used to remove dissolved solids) or cleaned by another government-approved method.
- **Artesian.** It came from a well that tapped an aquifer (a water-bearing rock formation) in which the water level is above that of the natural water table.

water before meals. One study at Agricultural University at Waginingen in the Netherlands showed drinking two glasses of water can make you feel less hungry when eating, possibly reducing your food intake and aiding weight loss.

Drink first, avoid thirst. Dehydration starts well before you feel thirsty, says Cochran. Once you feel thirsty, your body is essentially begging you to pour some liquid down your throat.

Frozen Foods

Warming Up to Healthy Eats

It's Super Bowl Sunday. You turn on the TV—with the remote control, of course—walk a few steps to the fridge and pull a frozen sausage pizza out of the freezer. Then you pop it in the microwave and, within seconds, have a mouth-watering 570-calorie gameday feast, with half of those calories coming from fat. Is this a great country or what?

Now consider the ancient Greeks. They had it tough. For starters, there was no Super Bowl. (What a shame the Denver Broncos and Buffalo Bills weren't around back then.) Rather, they had the Olympics. But they didn't have television, let alone ESPN, so they had to go to the stadium to see the games. Worst of all, though, was this: Their idea of frozen food involved hiking to the top of a high mountain, gathering some snow and ice, hiking back down and tossing it into a huge hole insulated with straw.

No wonder all those Greek guys they made statues of were thin.

The lesson: Being a sports fan hasn't changed much in a few thousand years. But refrigeration has revolutionized the way we live. "I'm totally convinced the freezer is the most cost-saving and time-saving device that anyone can make an investment in, especially for a single person," says Diane Wilke, R.D., a nutrition consultant in private practice in Columbus, Ohio.

But only if its powers are used for good.

Freeze, Mister

Frozen food doesn't just mean all that stuff in the cardboard boxes and plastic bags that you can find in your nearby grocery store. Yes, we'll be talking about that stuff in this chapter, too. But for right now, we're talking about food *you* make.

First of all, the stuff you make tastes a heck of a lot better than the stuff they make. Second, you have more control over the nutritional content of the stuff you make.

And it's not too hard to make your own frozen dinners. Every time you cook, pretend you're making enough to serve an Army mess hall. (Just forget about the creamed beef on toast.) Then break down all the leftovers into meal-size portions and throw them in the freezer, Wilke advises.

Some ideas:

Prepare plenty of pasta. Next time you make spaghetti, dump the entire box in with the boiling water. Eat what you want at that time, then freeze the rest with the sauce on it right in the casserole dish or in plastic bags. You can do the same thing with lasagna, manicotti or any other pasta dish. With baked pastas, make up two dishes. Then slice it up into individual servings and freeze it in freezer wrap. If you're going to eat it all within two to four weeks, you can use regular plastic wrap.

Grill burgers by the dozen. Make a mother lode, using lean beef or ground turkey. "If you're going to fire up the grill, don't just fix 2 hamburgers—fix 12," Wilke says. "My husband is chief pilot with an airline company

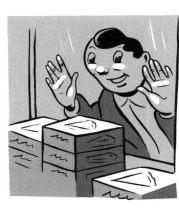

and my sons are both gone, so I'm all by myself. Some neighbors stopped over the other day. I had 12 hamburgers on the grill, and one of them asked who was coming for dinner. I said, 'Nobody. This is just what's going in the freezer.' " When the hamburgers cool, you can wrap them individually in freezer wrap or freezer resealable plastic storage bags and stack the wrapped burgers in your freezer. Then zap them in the microwave when you're ready to eat them.

No microwave? Then take them out of the plastic, wrap them in aluminum foil and heat them in the oven. If they come out too dry to eat on a bun, break them down and use the meat in stews, chilies or casseroles, says Nancy D. Berkoff of the Los Angeles Trade Technical College.

Don't loaf—cook extra. Next time you make meat loaf for dinner, make two and use ground turkey breast instead of beef, because it is a good low-fat alternative for this American classic. (Check the package label to make sure you purchase ground turkey breast because ground turkey made with the skin and dark meat can be very high in fat, Wilke warns.) Wrap the extra one in plastic or freezer wrap and toss it in the freezer. You also can cut up the meat loaf and wrap individual portions for meat loaf sandwiches.

Make lots when it's chili. You can't make too much chili—it's one of those immutable laws of nature. The same goes for chunky soups and stews. Store the extras in small containers. Note: Any food that has tomato in it has to be wrapped in plastic. It cannot be wrapped in foil because the acid in the tomato sauce will react with the foil and eat holes in it, says Rodale's Anita Hirsch.

Do the monster mash. Make a huge amount of mashed potatoes but use skimmed milk to save on fat and calories. Eat what you want, then store the rest in one-size portions in microwaveable plastic bags for future microwave magic.

A final note. When storing things, make sure to wrap them airtight in freezer resealable plastic storage bags, freezer wrap or foil, says Dr. Mona R. Sutnick of the American Dietetic Association. That avoids freezer burn and preserves the flavor, she says. Also, leave some room in the containers for the food to expand and write the freezing date on them. When you pull something out of your freezer, it's nice to know whether it's a few weeks old or a few years old. (For more information on how long foods can keep when frozen, see "Keeping It Cold" on page 42.)

Sealing in Nutrients

Because frozen vegetables are not fresh, they're not as good for you, right?

Wrong.

Frozen foods, especially vegetables and fruits, are nutritional powerhouses for two reasons. First, the freezing process locks in the vitamins and other nutrients. Some frozen fruits and vegetables may actually have slightly *more* nutrients than fresh batches because of less exposure to air or sunlight. Though the difference is slight, frozen blueberries, raspberries, green beans and broccoli may have more nutrients than fresh ones.

Second, we generally cook frozen foods in the microwave, and that's the number one cooking method to preserve nutrients, says Gertrude Armbruster, Ph.D., associate professor of nutritional sciences at Cornell University in Ithaca, New York.

Dr. Armbruster has compared the vitamin content of microwaved, steamed and boiled food. The microwaved food came out on top, followed by steamed.

"It has been known for some time that cooking vegetables in water in the conventional way results in vitamin losses," Dr. Armbruster says. "In microwave cooking it is not necessary to add this large body of water to cook vegetables to keep them from burning. The hypothesis is this should increase the nutrient retention."

Vegetables: Out in the Cold

You could hang out in the frozen food aisle for days. Just about everything imaginable comes frozen these days, from egg rolls to strawberry pies, but lots of the stuff is packed with salt and fat.

Frozen entrées, however, have made progress. Many frozen dinners are low fat and low salt. Problem is, when they cut out the fat and the salt, they also inexplicably cut out the vegetables, according to the Center for Science in the Public Interest. And most guys are struggling to get their five to nine servings a day.

A report on frozen entrées by the folks at the Center for Science in the Public Interest found 92 of 96 healthier, lower-fat, lower-salt frozen dinners supplied less than two half-cup servings of fruits or vegetables. More than a third—35 of the dinners—provided less than one-half cup, which is considered one serving.

The researchers picked the peas from the pasta and carrots from rice, and they were lenient, counting tomato sauce as a vegetable and those sugary, sloppy apple desserts as fruit. They found some interesting stuff.

- Healthy Choice's Chicken Francesca has only a tablespoon of asparagus and a tablespoon of red pepper.
- Lean Cuisine's Chicken à l'Orange with broccoli and rice had a tablespoon of broccoli and two teaspoons of carrots.

When you buy meals that don't even provide one serving of vegetables, you should make your own extra vegetables, says Wilke. For instance, eat your frozen dinner with a baked potato or stir up some frozen vegetables. If you eat a cup and a half of them, it counts as three vegetable servings.

Some low-fat (three grams or less per serving), low-sodium (less than 140 milligrams per serving) dinners that contain at least a cup of vegetables or fruit according to the Center for Science in the Public Interest include: Healthy Choice Zucchini Lasagna Entrée, Tyson Healthy Portion BBQ Chicken and Budget Gourmet Light and Healthy Yankee Pot Roast Dinner.

The Magic of Microwaving

If you have any natural curiosity whatsoever, the invention of the microwave oven turned your kitchen into an authentic science lab. The owner's manual quickly gathered dust as you tested the oven's powers day after day. There was the hot dog experiment. You and some buddies peered through the glass as the dog cooked. You took it out and slapped it onto a slice of bread. "Who wants it?" Everyone took a step back. You fed it to the dog. Spot didn't die. Conclusion: It's okay to eat micro dogs.

Today, our microwaves have lost their awe-inspiring nature. They're just one more thing in the kitchen. Thing is, most of us still don't have a clue how those gadgets work.

Worry not. Here's an explanation for just about everything you could possibly wonder about your microwave.

How does it cook food inside out? It doesn't. That's microwave folklore. This is how the oven works. It has a magnetron tube that converts electricity into microwaves. The waves travel throughout the oven. They pass through some things, such as glass, without heating it. They will bounce off other stuff, such as metal, causing arcing and possibly backfiring on the magnetron unit. And they are attracted to moist stuff, such as food.

The waves penetrate the food to the depth of about an inch. Waves make the food molecules rub against one another, creating friction, which creates heat. As the outer portion of the food heats up, heat travels inward.

Why can I only cook with particular materials?

As we said earlier, the microwaves react differently to different surfaces. You want to cook with something that the microwaves will pass through, such as glass, some plastics, ceramic, clay and paper, says Cornell University's Dr. Gertrude Armbruster. You want to stay away from metal because, as we said before, it reflects the waves away from the food and can make the waves arc, which can damage your microwave. Because recycled paper towels have metal fragments, you don't want to use them either, says Dr. Armbruster.

Why can't I turn it on unless something's inside? The microwaves need something to cook. If you run the oven without food inside, the rogue waves could damage your unit.

Why does it take longer to cook two potatoes than it does for one potato? Each thing you put in there sucks up waves. Basically, you have the same amount of waves with more stuff absorbing them. So it takes longer.

How do I get it to stop smelling like popcorn? First, clean it. Food splatters increase the cooking time because the food particles continue to cook every time you turn on the microwave. If wiping the interior with a damp cloth won't do the job, boil some water inside the unit to allow the steam to loosen up the grime, recommends Dr. Armbruster. Then wipe it down. To zap odors, boil a cup of water with a teaspoon of lemon juice. Then let it stand inside the oven for five minutes, she says.

Be a Smart Shopper

The frozen food aisle can be a bewildering place. If you rely solely on the photographs of sumptuous gourmet meals that grace most boxes, you're setting yourself up for major disappointment—and probably a few additional pounds.

Here are some things to look for.

Read the label. Not the whole thing. We know you're busy. But zoom in on the calories, sodium and fat content, suggests Hirsch. The terms "lower fat" and "lower sodium" are not the same thing as "low fat" and "low sodium." Lower only means it doesn't have as much as it used to.

Watch the portions. Many frozen entrées have cut down the number of fat grams by cutting down on the amount of food. The result: You're still a hungry man when you're done eating. Concentrate on the percent of calories that come from fat.

Supplement your supper. Even though their portions are skimpy, many dinners come with some type of sauce that's more filling than it looks. Still, you'll need to eat something else with the dinner to fill yourself up. Try baked potatoes, hot vegetables, salads, quick-cooking brown rice or whole-grain bread slices, recommends Hirsch.

Don't one-stop shop. Try single pasta and rice meals as well as the traditional kind that give you the meat, starch, vegetable and dessert all in the same box. You'll want to add more complex carbohydrates and vegetables to your diet and less meat, says Hirsch, if you want to cut fat and add fiber.

Desert big desserts. A gallon of ice cream can be dangerous. You take it out of the freezer, grab a spoon, sit in front of the TV with it and later realize you're out of ice cream. Instead, buy low-fat or nonfat frozen desserts in smaller portion sizes, says Hirsch. Popsicles are a good example. If you want to eat more than one, though, you'll have to keep getting up and going to the freezer to get it.

Canned Foods

Store Them for Convenience

Back in World War II in the First Infantry Division somewhere in North Africa, Fred Seward ate cold Spam in the dark with a sharpened spoon. The next night, he would eat Spam again. Same with the next. And the next.

It was the going Army joke during those hellish days whenever C rations were handed out: "Spam again?" But Seward knew the canned pork concoction was better than nothing. So he ate it. And ate it again.

Once he returned to the United States, he didn't touch Spam until nearly 50 years later. It was the same story with corned beef hash and orange marmalade. "Any canned food, if you have it day after day after day, becomes boring and monotonous and you will not touch it," says Seward, who now resides in Geneva, New York.

As for other foods that come canned—especially corn and peaches—Seward eats them heartily. They're convenient.

And convenience is canned food's main selling point. All the chopping, peeling and cooking has been done for you. If you come home from touch football feeling like a hungry piece of pulp—too hungry to sleep and too tired to eat—there's always that can of ravioli. Rip off the top, find a fork and you have dinner.

Some foods we would just never eat had our ancestors not had the foresight to invent canning: beans. The dried kind need to be soaked overnight.

"People who would not spend the time it takes to cook dried beans will use the cans. It's so convenient," says Dr. Mona R. Sutnick of the American Dietetic Association. "Beans are such good, nutritious food. They have a lot of the

same nutrients as meat, without the fat and cholesterol. And they're versatile. You can really do a lot with them whether it's soups or stews or chilies or salads."

Canned food's other claim to fame harkens back to your Boy Scout days—which, if you're lucky, is the last time you had to eat a lot of food from a can: Be prepared. Just in case Hurricane Elmer wipes out the utility poles in the entire county. Just in case a blizzard dumps enough snow to block access to a grocery store for a month. Just in case an earthquake swallows your refrigerator. According to the Canned Food Information Council in Chicago, this is what you should always have on hand—just in case.

- Canned fruit packed in its own juice (pears, mixed assortments, peaches)
- Canned meats and seafood packed in water or broth (tuna, chicken, crabmeat, salmon)
- Canned vegetables (corn, carrots, tomatoes, potatoes)
- Canned specialty food (chili, chow mein, Mexican dishes)
- Soups, including the low-fat and reduced-sodium varieties (vegetable, chicken noodle, stew)
- Beverages (condensed skim milk, fruit and vegetable juices)

You Can Do It

About 1,500 different foods come in cans, including 75 types of juices, 130 vegetable products and 100 soups and stews. That's a lot to chose from. Here's how to pick out the right stuff and cook it the right way so you can have a nutritious canned meal.

Drink the juice. When you buy a peach, the vitamins are in the peach. But when you buy a canned peach, only some of the vitamins are in the peach. The rest are in the liquid the peach is floating in. That's

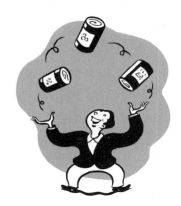

because nutrients will dissolve in water, says Dr. Sutnick.

You can get the most nutrients for your money by using the liquid from canned fruits and vegetables. And you don't have to drink it straight from the can. Here are some more palatable suggestions from Dr. Sutnick.

- Cook vegetables in the juice they come in.
- Use vegetable juice to make soup or stew.
- Put leftover fruit juice in ice cube trays and freeze it. You can eat it plain or put the cubes into drinks for extra flavor.
- Put fruit syrup on pancakes instead of maple syrup.

Pack it in water. You don't want to buy tuna that's packed in oil, because it has more fat and more calories than tuna packed in water. Even after you drain the oil, you're looking at three times as much fat and 50 percent more calories, according to researchers at the University of California, Berkeley. And you're getting less of the fish's healthy benefits. The healthy omega-3 fatty acids are oil soluble. When you drain the oil, you lose 15 to 25 percent of the omega-3's. You don't have the same problem with water-packed tuna.

Bone up on your calcium. If you want to boost your calcium intake, eat the bones from canned sardines and canned salmon. The bones will be soft from the processing. A three-ounce serving supplies as much calcium as a glass of milk.

Remember the good oil. When we think canned fish, we usually think tuna. On average, each of us eats about three pounds of it a year. You may, however, want to consider expanding your tastes. Canned salmon, sardines and herring have more omega-3's than tuna.

Sardines and herring can vary tremendously in their fat and caloric content because different packing companies use varying

Can Do Technology

Canned foods are preserved, yet they don't need preservatives. Here's how the food gets from the farm to your table.

1. The farmer grows it.
2. The food is shipped to a nearby canning plant.
3. Machines use high-pressure water sprays to wash the food.
4. More machines prepare the food. That means carrots are peeled and sliced, ears of corn are shucked, fruit is pitted and so on.
5. The food gets blanched to preserve flavor and texture and prevent spoilage.
6. Machines stuff the food into cans.
7. Machines dump water (which sometimes contains spices) into the cans.
8. The cans are vacuum sealed, cooked and then cooled.
9. They're shipped to the grocery store.

species and sizes of fish from different locations (those from colder waters have more fat). They can have anywhere from 2 to 20 grams of fat in three ounces. You need to read the label.

Watch the syrup. Look for fruit packed in its own juice or in light syrup. Heavy syrup packs more empty sugar calories than you need.

Watch the sodium. The National Academy of Sciences recommends we eat no more than 2,400 milligrams of sodium a day, the amount in one teaspoon of salt. The average American takes in close to 4,000 milligrams a day. And 75 percent of it comes from processed food.

Some soups have as much as 1,000 milligrams of salt per cup, so you need to read the label. Canned food manufacturers are putting out many reduced-salt products. Some include:

green beans, sliced beets, diced carrots, whole-kernel corn, sweet peas, mixed vegetables, garbanzo beans, tuna, salmon and soups. Here's how to understand the terms.

- Sodium-free. Less than 5 milligrams of sodium per serving.
- Very low sodium. Less than 35 milligrams per serving.
- Low sodium. 140 milligrams or less per serving.

Don't rinse it. Rinsing canned food will reduce the salt content, but it will also reduce its nutrient content. Unfortunately, the most heavily salted canned foods are soups, sauces, gravies and prepared foods, like pasta meals, which you couldn't or wouldn't rinse anyway. Dr. Sutnick suggests you look for low-salt or low-sodium versions of those products.

Just Add Taste

Some canned foods are overcooked and mushy. Some can be downright bland and boring. So what's a guy to do?

You need to get creative.

"Don't ask the food manufacturers to make it taste good. You're in charge of taste," says nutrition consultant Diane Wilke. "All you want is something that's basically healthy that is safe to eat. If it doesn't taste the way you like it, then you modify it to make it taste better."

So add some zest to canned foods by adding salsa, ketchup, garlic, onions or nonfat Italian dressing.

And don't overcook the peas—or any other canned foods. Remember, they're already cooked. You only need to warm them up. It only takes a couple of minutes in a sauce pan or microwave to get them ready to eat. Techni-cally, you can eat them straight from the can.

In the Can

How healthy is that stuff on your pantry shelf? Take a look.

Product	Sodium (mg.)	Fat (g.)
Baked beans with beef (1 cup)	1,264	9.2
Baked beans with franks (1 cup)	1,105	16.9
Baked beans with pork (1 cup)	1,048	3.9
Heinz Vegetarian Beans (½ cup)	480	0.5
Chef Boyardee Cheese Tortellini (1 cup)	770	1
Chef Boyardee Spaghetti and Meatballs (1 cup)	940	9
Del Monte Sloppy Joe Sauce (¼ cup)	680	0
La Choy Beef Chow Mein (1 cup)	760	1.5
La Choy Chicken Fried Rice (1 cup)	1,020	1
La Choy Chicken Sweet and Sour	660	2.5
Mary Kitchen Corned Beef Hash (1 cup)	930	24
Beef noodle soup (½ cup)	920	2.5
Campbell's Bean with Bacon soup (½ cup)	890	5
Campbell's California-Style Vegetable soup (½ cup)	850	1

We're not saying you should plop cans of corn, beans and peas with the lids ripped off on your kitchen table for dinner. We're saying that if you want to save time, you can find ways to use them without even heating them. Make a cold salad out of them. Throw some canned carrots, kidney beans and lima beans together with a marinade. Or mix canned collard greens with some onion and vinegar.

Here are some other ways to throw together a quick canned food meal, according to the Canned Food Information Council. Dr. Sutnick recommends that you always look for the light, low-sodium, low-fat versions of canned foods you choose.

Mix it up. Mix canned fruit with plain nonfat yogurt.

Product	Sodium (mg.)	Fat (g.)
Campbell's Chicken with Rice (½ cup)	830	2.5
Campbell's Golden Corn soup (½ cup)	730	3.5
Chicken noodle soup (½ cup)	950	2
Cream of asparagus soup (½ cup)	910	7
Cream of celery soup (½ cup)	900	7
Cream of chicken soup (½ cup)	890	8
Cream of mushroom soup (½ cup)	870	7
Manhattan clam chowder (½ cup)	910	0.5
New England clam chowder (½ cup)	980	2.5
Tomato bisque soup (½ cup)	900	3
Green beans (½ cup)	170	0.1
Kidney beans (1 cup)	873	0.9
Lima beans (1 cup)	809	0.4
Mixed vegetables (½ cup)	122	0.2
Mushrooms (½ cup)	440	0
Yellow corn (½ cup)	0	0.8

First fruit. You could pay a lot more money for pretty, uniform pear halves. And there are times when you should. If you're cooking up a special dinner, you might want to open up a can of pretty pear halves and arrange them in a pretty bowl.

But if you're just going to rip off the top of the can and jam your fork into the first pear it comes in contact with, there's no need to pay for elegance. Get the cheaper kind.

Same with tuna. There's only one thing to look for in tuna. We already told you about it. You don't want it packed in oil. Other than that, it doesn't matter what you buy. Light meat, dark meat. That's a personal preference, but it won't affect your health, says Dr. Sutnick.

Same with the size of the chunks. If you're going to mash it up, don't go wasting your cash on solid tuna, which costs more. Get the flaked kind. Hey, they've done half the work for you already.

The rule applies to any canned item. "Don't buy fancier than you're going to use," says Dr. Sutnick.

Dump it. Dump canned vegetables into various canned soups.

Top it off. Use canned peaches or blueberries on top of low-fat pound cake.

Garnish it. Place canned pineapple rings around various meats and poultry.

Toss it. Toss cooked and cooled rotini or pasta shells with drained canned tomatoes, canned carrots, canned mushrooms and a vinaigrette dressing.

Shop Smart

Canned food is cheap, but there are some things you don't need to go wasting your money on. One of them is elegance. Two canned items come to mind: fruit and tuna.

On the Shelf

As long as it stays in the can and the can is undamaged, the stuff could probably last forever. But you don't want to take chances. The Canned Food Information Council recommends you use the canned foods within a year or donate them to a local food drive.

Don't store cans above 80°F. Also, beware of cans that look damaged. If the vacuum seal has been ruptured, the food has not been preserved. And it can make you really sick, so watch out for swelling or leaks.

Some hissing when the can is opened is normal because it's vacuum-packed. But if the can hisses loudly or spurts, the food might be spoiled, according to the council.

Pastas and Grains

How to Better Your Bread

In ancient Rome white bread was revered as the food of the gods. The concept was so ingrained that the politically powerful mixed chalk in with their flour to ensure their loaves were as pasty as possible.

Lots of things have changed since then. Rome fell. (For lack of Wonder Bread? You be the judge.) And the idea that white bread is the ultimate nutritional powerhouse has been relegated to the dungheap of history, somewhere between that wacky old flat-earth theory and the even more frightening notion from the 1970s that men could look fetching in lime-green leisure suits.

Why is dark bread better? It's the same reason whole-wheat pasta is better than pasta made from white flour. It's the same reason that brown rice is better than white. And it's the same reason that oatmeal is better than Cream of Wheat. It all depends on what part of the grain is used to make the food.

Planting the Seed for Good Health

Grains are seeds that come from grasses. You can think of them pretty much as anything you've seen waving in the wind while driving along some desolate country road: wheat, corn, oats, barley, millet, rice and rye.

To understand why some parts of the grain are better than others, you first need to know the parts of the grain.

- Endosperm. The largest part of the grain but the least nutritional. It does contain starch, some protein and a few B vitamins.

- Germ. The smallest part of the grain and the most nutritionally concentrated. It contains protein, oils and the B vitamins thiamin, riboflavin, niacin and pyridoxine. It also has vitamin E and the minerals magnesium, zinc, potassium and iron.
- Bran. The grain's fiber powerhouse. This coating around the endosperm contains B vitamins, zinc, calcium, potassium, phosphorus, magnesium and some other minerals. A bowl of high-bran cereal with milk has as much potassium as a medium banana.

Though the endosperm barely has any nutritional value, it's refined (the process of removing the bran and germ) and ground up to make the white flour that is a key component in white bread and pale pasta. The government requires manufacturers to enrich such refined products with thiamin, riboflavin, niacin and iron.

But products that are made with the other parts of the grain—oat bran muffins, whole-wheat bread, wheat germ, brown rice—are naturally more nutritious.

About now, you're probably wondering if you're ever allowed to eat white bread and pale pasta again. The answer is yes. You just want to eat more of the dark stuff, too, says Jane Folkman, R.D., spokesperson for the Massachusetts Dietetic Association in Boston.

The most important reason to eat a lot of whole grains is fiber. Fiber helps you avoid cancer, lower your cholesterol and keep your digestive tract running smoothly. But fiber grams do not add up easily. One bagel has about 0.5 gram, a slice of whole-wheat bread 1.5 grams and a cup of enriched spaghetti has 2.2 grams. So you can see why nutritionists want you to eat 6 to 11 servings of grains and cereals a day.

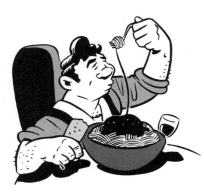

"If you eat more foods such as brown rice and whole-wheat pasta, it's a lot easier to meet that recommendation,"

says Neva Cochran of the American Dietetic Association. Grains are also low in fat and high in complex carbohydrates.

Weighing In

But can't too many grain products such as pasta and bread make you fat?

No. It's true starchy foods can raise insulin levels abnormally high in about 10 to 20 percent of the population. That makes them more susceptible to heart disease, but it doesn't make them fat. Many such people have insulin problems because they are already overweight, because they don't exercise or because their genes made them that way.

Going strictly by the numbers, it would seem that eating more pasta and other grain products would help with weight loss. Grains are carbohydrates, which have four calories per gram. Fat has nine calories per gram—if we ate the same amount of food but cut the fat and increased the carbohydrates, it would make sense that we would lose weight.

The problem is that we haven't done that. Between 1978 and 1990 Americans cut their average intake of dietary fat from 36 percent to 34 percent of our total calories. Basically, that's one less teaspoon of butter a day. But we gained weight.

Why? It wasn't the switch from fatty meats to nonfatty pastas and grains. We got fatter because we ate more during the same time period, increasing our daily calories. And we began exercising less, says Gerald Reaven, M.D., professor emeritus of medicine at Stanford University School of Medicine. He says it is unclear which factor is most responsible for our collective weight gain.

"It's the total number of calories you eat and what your caloric expenditure is. So if you run five miles a day, you'll use up more calories than if you don't run five miles a day. It's a function of caloric intake and caloric expenditure," Dr. Reaven says.

Pasta is not fattening unless you eat six bowls of spaghetti when you usually would eat only one. Try to follow the Food Guide Pyramid. Six to 11 servings of pastas and grains really isn't that much when you consider what counts as a serving—one slice of bread, a half-cup of cooked cereal or a half-cup of rice. Some specialty shop bagels are so big they equal four servings. And a typical serving of spaghetti will count as three.

The Bread of Life

Different breads have different amounts of fiber, varying between one and over three grams per slice. Read the label to find high-fiber breads.

Also, like we said before, look for breads made from whole grains. That means the bread should have the word "whole" somewhere in its title. For instance, whole-wheat bread has more zinc, magnesium, fiber and other nutrients than refined white bread. The refining process strips those nutrients. Wheat bread usually has twice the fiber of white bread. White bread, however, is enriched with iron and B vitamins—thiamin, niacin and riboflavin.

If you're looking to buy wheat bread, be careful to read the labels. Some breads have wheat-sounding titles but are really made with refined flour. To make sure you're getting whole wheat, look for "whole wheat" or another whole grain as the first ingredient on the label, says Cochran.

It's okay to eat other stuff like French bread, rye, pumpernickel, sourdough and English muffins, because they are packed with healthy complex carbohydrates, says Cochran. But don't fool yourself into thinking you're getting whole grains. You might get a pinch of the whole rye seed with your bread, but most of it is made from refined flour. And the dark color of pumpernickel usually comes from coloring.

Bread can dry out in the fridge. Wrap English muffins, pitas, bagels and other breads tightly with plastic wrap and store them at room temperature or in the freezer.

Using Your Noodle

They are proud of their pasta over there in Europe. So proud, in fact, that they openly bicker about who invented it. One crowd argues that Marco Polo brought the initially Chinese dish back to Europe after he visited Kubla Khan. But Italians don't buy it. A few years back, they decided pasta was so important it should have its very own museum. At this National Museum of Pasta Foods they argue that Italians served noodles at least a hundred years before Marco Polo even thought about China. It just seemed new because the Chinese were serving pasta differently.

Another thing they tell you at this museum: Whatever you do, don't overcook the noodles. With that in mind, here's what you need to know in order to eat pasta like an Italian.

Get in shape. There are more than 300 different shapes that fall into five basic categories. There are long, round noodles such as spaghetti and angel hair, and long, flat ones such as linguine and lasagna. There's the tube variety such as ziti, macaroni and penne, and the corkscrew type such as fusilli and rotini. Finally, there's the potluck category that includes everything that doesn't fit into the above. That includes those wagon wheels, the ABCs in alphabet soup and specialty pastas shaped like chili peppers, bicycles and even sex organs. The various shapes go well with various sauces.

Go for flour power. Look for pasta that's made from a good flour. In most cases, you want something made from 100 percent semolina (ground durum wheat). It's what's known as a hard flour. It won't absorb much water when cooked, so it will always turn out firm. It's good with a variety of sauces from light sauces made with olive oil to heavy, chunky sauces. Some refrigerated pastas are instead made from regular bread flour (ground up endosperm), which is known as a soft flour. If you like limp pasta, that's fine. But be forewarned: No matter what you do, it will never turn out firm. Asian noodles offer an expanded selection in tastes because they are made with so many varied sources: buckwheat, rice, mung beans, potato starch and sweet potatoes.

Know your dough. The pasta you buy at the grocery store is usually what's known as dry pasta. It's fine for almost all occasions, but if you want to treat yourself, try refrigerated fresh or soft pasta available at specialty shops and some supermarkets. It cooks faster, tastes doughier and usually costs more dough. It also is usually made with egg, which means it has more cholesterol. It will only keep in the refrigerator for a day or two, so plan to cook it up quickly.

Eat Popeye pasta. Some pastas have ingredients other than flour, and that's what makes some nutritionally different from others. Some types contain egg, which means as much as 145 milligrams of cholesterol per serving. Others have some spinach, and almost all semolina products are enriched with extra nutrients. Spinach and wheat pastas can be a good way to boost your nutrient intake. For example, one cup of cooked spinach spaghetti has 42 milligrams of calcium, 87 milligrams of magnesium, 81 milligrams of potassium and 151 milligrams of phosphorus. One cup of regular, cooked spaghetti, in comparison, has 10 milligrams of calcium, 25 milligrams of magnesium, 44 milligrams of potassium and 76 milligrams of phosphorus.

Keep it in the dark. You can keep dried, uncooked pasta in a cool, dry cupboard for up to one year. You can refrigerate cooked pasta for three to five days. The cooked pasta will continue to absorb flavor from the sauce unless you store it separately.

Follow directions. To avoid clumpy pasta, make sure you give it enough water. Boil four to six quarts of water per pasta pound. Also, stir often. In terms of cooking time, there's really no magical advice. Follow the package directions, according to Donna Chowning Reid, director of communications for the National Pasta Association in Arlington, Virginia. Each manufacturer has tested its pasta to determine the optimum cooking time, and each pasta is different. If you're not the clock-watching type, you can nibble a piece every so often. Pasta is done when it's firm yet cooked all the way through.

Converting to Rice

It's been around since 2,800 B.C., and next to spaghetti, rice is probably one of the easiest things to cook.

It comes in three different sizes. Long-grain rice is four times as long as it is wide, compared to short grain, which is round. Long-grain rice comes out fluffy and easy to separate. Medium grain is more moist and tender, and short grain sticks together after cooking—good for rolling sushi.

Rice comes in many varieties, but most familiar are brown and white. Brown rice provides more fiber, vitamin E, phosphorus and calcium than white rice. But most white rice is enriched and provides more thiamin and iron than brown rice. Here are some ways to spice it up.

Try something new. Other varieties of rice include converted, aromatic and wild. Converted rice is Uncle Ben's. It has been steamed under pressure before milling, which returns some of the bran's nutrients without keeping the bran intact. The rice turns out firm and fluffy. Aromatic rice is the term used to describe any variety of rice that has a strong, nutty aroma. Wild rice is not really a member of the rice family but the seed of an aquatic grass. It has more protein than white rice and has a nutty flavor.

Keep a lid on it. Once opened, uncooked rice should be stored in a tightly sealed container in a cool, dry place. The shelf life for brown rice is shorter than white. The bran layers of brown rice have oil that can go rancid, so the U.S.A. Rice Council suggests storing it in the refrigerator. It will keep in the fridge for about six months.

Go slow. When cooking rice, slowly add it to boiling water. Make sure there's enough water for the rice to float freely. And of course, follow the package directions.

Bagel Blunders

All you wanted was a quick breakfast. Instead, you got a quick trip to the emergency room to get your finger stitched up.

"People are often embarrassed to tell you," says Mark Smith, M.D., chairman of the Department of Emergency Medicine at Washington Hospital Center and clinical professor of emergency medicine at The George Washington University School of Medicine and Health Sciences, both in Washington, D.C. "We noticed that it was sufficiently common that we identified it as a syndrome. You usually get one or two people a weekend."

George Washington University hospital doctors were seeing so many bagel injuries that they did some research. They called some bagel stores, and they came up with some cutting-edge advice.

Get a grip. Some bagel shops or kitchen supply stores sell devices that will hold your bagel steady as you slice. They keep your fingers out of the knife's way.

Make a lateral move. Put the bagel flat on the table and slice parallel to the table. Though your hand should be out of harm's way, not too many experts are fond of this method. This is no time to get cocky.

Stay above the fray. With your thumb and index finger, hold the bagel perpendicular to the table. Your thumb and index finger should be shaped like an upside down U. For instance, if you're holding the bagel in your left hand, your thumb should be toward you, to the left. Put the knife edge in the space between the thumb and index finger and cut down. "This way your fingers are above the knife and it's hard to cut yourself," Dr. Smith says.

Cereals

The Breakfast of Champions

Ask most guys why they don't eat breakfast and odds are they'll tell you they don't have time. What they really mean is that they hit the snooze button instead of getting up when the alarm goes off. And when it comes to breakfast, if you snooze, you lose. But you don't have to roll out of bed an hour early to make pancakes from scratch. Just reach for a box of cereal, the lazy man's grub.

"Cereal to me is one of the easiest things in the world, not just in terms of making it but also in terms of cleaning up before I leave the house," says an admittedly lazy John Stanton, Ph.D., food marketing professor at St. Joseph's University in Philadelphia. "It's one stinking bowl. I don't even need to turn the stove on."

Actually, it's so easy, it doesn't seem possible that it's allowed to be good for you. But it is. Of all the things you can eat in the morning, Dr. Stanton says, cereal is one of the best choices.

Hot cereal has most of the same benefits as cold, but there's one hitch. It involves either using your stove or your microwave. "They just take longer. That's the only problem. I could eat oatmeal every day if someone would get up and make it for me," Dr. Stanton says.

Bulk in a Bowl

Men need fiber. Doctors recommend we get between 25 and 35 grams of fiber a day. That's hard to do unless you're a musk ox. Most men only get 10 to 12 grams of fiber a day. Cereal is a quick and easy way to add some bulk to your diet.

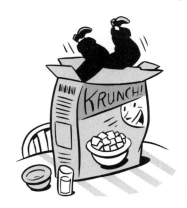

Elizabeth Somer, R.D., author of *Food and Mood*, recommends picking a cereal that has at least two grams of fiber per serving. Cereals made primarily from corn, wheat, oats or rice—particularly bran cereals such as Kellogg's All-Bran—have as much as 14 grams of fiber per serving. Then again, some, like General Mills's Boo Berry, have none. So you have to check nutrition information on the box. Remember, that's what it's there for.

Just because some cereals will fill half of your daily fiber requirement doesn't mean you need to torture yourself by eating stuff you think tastes like the sole of your running shoe. And you need to get your fiber from more than just your cereal.

"People know that they are supposed to eat more fiber, but they think that eating a bran cereal is the answer to their fiber needs. What they need to do is eat a high-fiber diet," Somer says. "A high-fiber diet that contains lots of fruits, vegetables, whole grains and legumes provides a blend of different fibers that in turn promote health and the prevention of heart disease, diabetes, high blood pressure, cancer and more."

Eating at least two grams of fiber a day will help lower your cholesterol, and eating 25 grams a day will lower your risk of colon cancer by 31 percent. Colon cancer is the third-most prevalent and fatal cancer in U.S. men. A high-fiber diet lowers your risk of getting it by decreasing the time waste sits around in the colon.

Many cereals also are crammed with vitamins. Most provide at least 10 percent of some of your vitamin and mineral needs. Some, such as Total, offer 100 percent of the recommended Daily Value for nine vitamins, iron and zinc.

Not only do they have good stuff, many cereals also are lacking in the bad stuff—fat. Most have only two grams or less per serving, although oat-based cereals and granolas usually have more. As a rule, look for cereals that have two grams of fat or less, says Somer. Besides clogging your arteries, a high-calorie, fat-laden meal can make you tired, she says. And that's the last sensation you need when heading for the office.

When picking out cereal, here are two other key things to look for.

• Sugar. Keep it to four grams or less per serving, suggests Somer. If the cereal has fruit in it, you can allow for more. Just remember what fruit is. Froot Loops do not contain fruit. Raisin Bran does.

• Protein. Try for at least three grams per serving, says Somer. The protein will perk up your brain, giving you peak mental performance through the morning. It also will quiet your stomach through those morning meetings. No one wants to be the guy whose "grrring" tummy gets everyone's attention.

Eat Early, Eat Less

It doesn't matter how much he knows about nutrition. If John Stanton, Ph.D., didn't eat breakfast, he'd be scooping high-fat peanut butter into his mouth. That's his vice.

And the food marketing professor at St. Joseph's University in Philadelphia suspects other people succumb to similar pitfalls. But their vice might be jelly doughnuts, chocolate chip cookies or potato chips. Fat. Fat. And more fat.

That explains the results of one of Dr. Stanton's studies. He found those who eat breakfast—regardless of the kind of breakfast—have lower cholesterol levels than those who rush off to work hungry. "By skipping breakfast, people obviously are hungry during the day," Dr. Stanton says. "They seek to make up the missing calories in their day by picking high-calorie choices. And those high-calorie choices are usually high-fat choices."

Getting in the Habit

It doesn't matter that it takes less than a minute to make a bowl of cereal. Some people just need a little help to get in the breakfast habit. Well, let's make that a lot of people. About a quarter of the population skips breakfast. But Dr. Stanton has some tips that may make morning eating easier.

Eat what you like. Stocking your shelf with cereals you like will increase your chance of eating them. If you buy one brand after another that tastes like cardboard, chances are you'll continue to skip breakfast, Dr. Stanton says. "Most of us do not believe we're put on this earth to live like monks in hair shirts. Food should have some pleasure to it," he says.

Make it interesting. Corn Flakes again? If you eat the same thing day after day, you're going to get bored. So stock your cereal shelf with different kinds of cereal. Then you can switch to Cinnamon Toast Crunch when Corn Flakes get boring, Dr. Stanton says.

Don't be fooled. It's happened to the best of us. There it is, beckoning you from the supermarket shelf: the most scrumptious-looking picture of a bowl of cereal you've ever seen. You throw the box in the cart. Then when you eat it the next day, it tastes exactly like the picture—cardboard. The result: a cereal cupboard full of once-poured cereal boxes. According to The First Really Important Survey of American Habits by Mel Poretz and Barry Sinrod, 6 percent of the respondents had more than seven boxes gathering dust in the kitchen. Another 19 percent had at least five or six. If you want to avoid being part of this statistic, ask your friends what they've tried or look for consumer guides that feature taste ratings on cereals to give you an idea of what's really good.

Snacks

Go Ahead—Eat between Meals

We know about three-quarters of you snack during the day. Some of you eat something nutritious such as fruit. Most of you, however, crave something really salty and crunchy, like potato chips. Come evening, you head for the fridge for ice cream. And most of you care more about taste than nutrition.

All of which leads us to this piece of wisdom: If we told you to give up potato chips, you wouldn't read this chapter.

So we won't. Instead, we'll help you solve that nutrition-versus-taste conflict researchers say you're having. The conflict is simple: We prefer potato chips to a banana. We wish we preferred a banana to chips. How then can we unclog our arteries with those lard-laden snacks staring us in the face?

Actually, it's not that hard. We just need to follow some simple rules.

Eat Early and Often

Here's exactly what you want to hear. You should snack. Forget what your parents told you about snacking between meals. Studies now show it's good for you.

Researchers at Trinity College Medical School in Dublin, Ireland, found that men's cholesterol is influenced by how many meals they eat a day. But it's not what you think. It turns out, the more frequent, smaller meals or snacks you eat, the better your cholesterol level.

Men who ate six meals instead of three—but otherwise had the same nutrient intake—

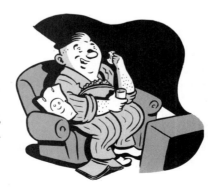

lowered their cholesterol. The researchers noted that frequent meal eating may be more effective at lowering cholesterol than changing to a low-fat diet, though eating low-fat snacks would help even more.

Snacking also can help you lose weight, says Maria Simonson, Sc.D., Ph.D., director of the Health, Weight and Stress Clinic at Johns Hopkins Medical Institutions in Baltimore. Your body can only use so many calories at one time. So when you stuff yourself three times a day, you're likely to store some of it as fat. If you spread out the same number of calories during five meals, you're more likely to burn the food for energy, Dr. Simonson says.

For similar reasons, people who snack also end up having more mental and physical energy. When you eat a huge lunch, the blood rushes to your stomach and away from your brain, causing your afternoon slump. (Isn't science wonderful? It even has an explanation for why Homer Simpson falls asleep at his nuclear power plant console all the time.) When you eat numerous small meals, you avoid the slump, says registered dietitian Elizabeth Somer.

To get the most out of snacking, you should eat every three to four hours, says Somer. Then there's no reason to have huge meals.

Snacking Strategies

You know fat is bad. And some snacks are almost all fat. Take the typical potato chip—or 15 of them, which is how many are in an ounce. Those 15 chips pack a total of ten grams of fat. But food manufacturers are coming out with more and more low-fat and nonfat snacks. There's everything from pretzels to potato chips to cakes. Granted, some of them taste, well, funny, but taste and selection are improving.

You can obtain a free catalog of nonfat snacks by calling Fatwise, a nonfat-snack distribution company, at (908) 862-3443.

Here are some ways to keep eating stuff that tastes good without making you fat, says Jayne Hurley, R.D., senior nutritionist at the Center for Science in the Public Interest in Washington, D.C., and a writer for the *Nutrition Action Healthletter*.

Bend your taste to pretzels. They are almost always low-fat because they are baked, not fried. Most have less than a gram of fat per ounce. A few, however, should be avoided. Combos Pepperoni Pizza snacks, for instance, have seven grams of fat per one-ounce serving.

The problem with pretzels is that they have a lot of salt, about 400 to 600 milligrams for every ounce. If you hate unsalted pretzels, try scraping off some of the salt on regular pretzels to lower your intake.

Other naturally low-fat snacks include air-popped popcorn and baked tortilla or potato chips.

Meet them halfway. If potato chips are what you're after but you can't stomach even the best nonfat chip, try Ruffles Reduced Fat or Pringles Right Crisps. They are not low-fat by any means with roughly seven grams of fat per ounce, but they are much lower than those with ten grams per ounce and taste about the same.

Don't be fooled. Listen to these words: multigrain chips, carrot chips, sweet potato chips. Sound healthy? They're not. Terra Sweet Potato chips, made from vegetables, have seven grams of fat per serving. A serving of Hain's Carrot Chips packs nine grams of fat but only offers the equivalent of one twenty-fifth of a carrot.

Squeeze in some fruit. Instead of

What's in This Stuff?

Here are the fat and caloric contents of some snacks.

Product (1 oz., unless otherwise indicated)	Calories	Fat (g.)
Betty Crocker Bugles Corn Snacks (1⅓ cups)	160	7
Chex Mix Traditional (⅔ cup)	130	3.5
Corn chips	153	8.8
Fritos Original Corn Chips	160	10
Nabisco Cheese Nips (29 crackers)	150	6
Planters Cheese Balls	150	10
Orville Redenbacher's Natural Microwave Popcorn (1 cup)	30	11
Pop Secret Movie Theater Butter Light Popcorn (1 cup)	25	6
Pop Secret Premium Microwave Popcorn (1 cup)	170	12
Pork skins	154	8.9
Eagle Ripples Natural Potato Chips	160	10
Lays Original Hickory BBQ Potato Chips	150	10
Pringles Original	160	11
Tortilla chips	142	7.4
Wise Genuine Texas Bar-B-Q Potato Chips	150	10
Eagle Mini Bites (¾ cup)	110	1
Combos Cheddar Cheese Pretzels	130	5
Keebler Knots (7 pretzels)	120	1
Wheat-based sesame sticks	153	10.4

tempting yourself with greasy snacks, make sure more nutritious foods are staring you down when your stomach grumbles, says Dr. Simonson. Take fruit and low-calorie bagels or pretzels to work. Put them on your kitchen table so when you wander in looking for something to eat, they'll be the first thing you see.

Oils

Extend the Olive Branch

You can get about 40 percent of your daily calories from fat and dramatically cut your risk of heart disease. Sound too good to be true? That's because it is. Like most things in life, you need to read the fine print when it comes to the Mediterranean diet.

Yes, the traditional Mediterranean eating plan gets about 40 percent of its calories from fat, primarily from olive oil. And, yes, those who feast on Mediterranean fare are among those who have the lowest risk of heart disease. But that doesn't mean men in the United States should start cooking chicken wings and french fries in olive oil if they want to live longer.

You see, it's not just the olive oil. We'd have to make a few other changes as well.

The Mediterranean people doctors have studied pushed plows around for a living; we sit in chairs and lay on couches. It took some of the Mediterranean folks anywhere from a week to a month to consume three ounces of meat— less than most of us eat in one day. They ate a lot of vegetables; we eat precious few.

"The good health of the Mediterranean population is almost certainly not just because of consumption of olive oil," says Harvard University's Dr. Walter C. Willett. "It's because of regular daily consumption of large amounts of fruits and vegetables and low amounts of animal products."

Saturated Fat: The Hydrogen Bomb

History has shown that with a healthy diet, olive oil is a good choice. But lots of other oils can be added to your diet to replace the unhealthy fat. If you want your body to be a well-oiled machine, you should know the difference between the two main families of fat that oils belong to. You've probably heard these terms a million times, but if you still don't know what makes some fats saturated and others unsaturated, don't worry. It has to do with hydrogen atoms.

What you really need to know can be summed up in one simple phrase: Jackson Browne was wrong. His debut album was named *Saturate Before Using*. When it comes to fat, the opposite is true. Here's why.

• Saturated fat clogs your arteries. Avoid it whenever possible. Most often found in animal products such as meats and butter, saturated fat is usually solid at room temperature. There are only three vegetable oils on the saturated list: coconut, palm and palm kernel oil. So stay away from them.

• Unsaturated fats are a bit more complicated. There are two kinds—monounsaturated and polyunsaturated. The monounsaturated group includes olive, peanut and canola oils, while corn, safflower and sesame oils belong to the polyunsaturated family.

The Poly versus Mono Debate

Over the years doctors have wavered in their recommendations concerning whether polyunsaturated or monounsaturated fats are better for you. When it comes to cholesterol levels, it seems there's not much difference between either type of oil, says Christopher Gardner, Ph.D., a research fellow at the Stanford Center for Research in Disease Prevention.

Some studies, though, have shown that polyunsaturated oils cause tumors in animals. "There's no evidence

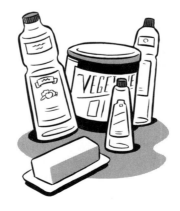

yet that it also applies to humans. But that has to make you a little bit cautious," Dr. Willett warns.

Of the various monounsaturated oils, there's really no evidence that one works better than the others. Some doctors say you should pick the most highly unsaturated oil you can find. Dr. Willett sides with olive oil, because people have consumed it for thousands of years with no ill effects.

Olive, canola and peanut are all highly monounsaturated.

Like a Virgin

If you're going to switch to olive oil, you need to learn some lingo. It will come in handy next time you're standing next to a beautiful woman in the oil aisle at the grocery store. When she asks, "What's extra virgin?" you do not—repeat—not answer, "It's made from the remains of a woman who was flung into a volcano to appease the gods."

Like the intelligent man you are, you will explain the differences between the various types of olive oils. And if you're smooth enough, you'll charm her into coming over to your place for dinner.

But you can't impress if you don't know. So pay attention as Arlene Wanderman, publicist for the International Olive Oil Council in New York City, explains the subtle differences. First of all, don't get hung up on how the olives are pressed.

Back in the old days some were pressed just once, others numerous times. Today, it's all done the same way. What matters is how acidic the olives are.

What follows is a primer on the various kinds of olive oils. Memorize it, and you can start planning that romantic dinner.

• Extra virgin. This is the most expensive and highest quality olive oil you can buy. It's called extra virgin because it's pure. The olives are handpicked at optimum ripeness, so their

oil produces a flavor that's known as perfect in olive oil connoisseur circles. It has a low acidity level—less than 1 percent acidity per 100 grams.

• Virgin. Somewhat inferior to extra virgin, virgin oil is not sold much in the United States. It has a slightly higher acidity level than extra virgin. That doesn't mean it will burn your tongue. It means the oil has slight imperfections in flavor and taste.

• Plain. When a bottle just says "olive oil," it means it's a blend of virgin oil and oil considered to be too acidic and too imperfect. It may cost less than other olive oils, but the cheaper price may be at the cost of good taste since olive oil connoisseurs say it lacks the flavor of other olive oils. The olives were most likely harvested by machine. They may have been picked too early. Or too late. Whatever happened in the harvesting process, the oil had to be refined and then blended with virgin oil, a process that olive oil connoisseurs say leaves it lacking in flavor.

• Unfiltered. Used mostly in Europe and by olive oil connoisseurs in the United States, unfiltered oil is a really strong extra virgin oil that looks cloudy and has small olive pieces floating through it.

• Light. That doesn't mean it has fewer calories. It means it has a mild flavor. Light oil has been filtered and refined. It's designed for people who want to use olive oil for health reasons but don't like the way it tastes.

Within those categories, olive oils still vary in taste and color. You basically have to try a bunch to see which ones you like.

Wanderman suggests keeping a bottle of extra virgin and a bottle of plain olive oil around the house. Use the plain olive oil for cooking, sautéing and frying. You wouldn't want to cook with expensive extra virgin because much of its flavor would evaporate.

You'll want to use the extra virgin as a seasoning. "I use it in salads. I use it on vegetables. I drizzle it over fish or meat. I use it like I would a condiment," Wanderman says.

Spices

There's a Whole Lot of Shaking Going On

You've been captured by a medieval king who doesn't like the way you look. He plans to burn you at the stake. But just to amuse himself, he decides to play a game. His servant dumps a dab of salt, a dab of pepper, a dab of dill and a dab of dried-up garlic onto a table. If you pick his favorite spice, he'll not only set you free but he'll let you take the fairest maiden and a pound of that spice with you. But if you choose wrong, he'll let his sadistic servant Ratsloth torture you for a year before he burns you to death.

Choose carefully. The *Jeopardy* theme is almost over.

Got your answer?

Okay, we'll give you a clue. Forget about the king's taste buds. There's only one spice on the table.

Your answer: pepper.

You see, technically, those dried-up garlic flakes you shake onto bread aren't spices. They're dehydrated vegetable seasonings. Neither is dill. It's an herb—the leafy part of a plant that grows in mild climates. Or salt. It's a combination of two elements—sodium and chlorine.

But hardly anyone knows the difference. So the spice industry has kidnapped a whole bunch of seasonings that technically are not spices and called them spices anyway. For the record, spices originally referred to plants that grew somewhere in the tropics. But if you call anything you shake on top of food a spice, it's not like somebody's going to flambé you for your faux pas.

The Spice of Life

You can, however, get burned at the dinner table if your idea of spicing your food stops at putting out the salt and pepper shakers. Your body only needs about a quarter-teaspoon of salt a day; most of us eat ten times that much.

Cutting down on the fat and salt in food does not condemn you to live the rest of your days in the Village of the Bland. By acquainting yourself with the little jars, bottles and tins in the spice section of your local supermarket, you can actually make your food taste better.

Make it potent. Salt usually brings out the flavor of other spices. So if you eliminate it entirely, you'll need something really strong to take its place. Curry powder, garlic, onion and black pepper (made from a dried berry called a peppercorn and with no relation to sweet and hot peppers) fit that description, says Rodale's Anita Hirsch. Garlic has other pluses besides making food taste better. According to scientific research, it can lower blood pressure and cholesterol, aids digestion and may even help fight cancer.

Dehydrated garlic and onion both come in different forms: powdered, granulated, ground, minced, chopped and sliced. If you only want to taste garlic on your food, the powdered or granulated kinds work best. If you want to see and feel the garlic or onion on your food, buy minced, chopped or sliced. Though you wouldn't want to use garlic on desserts or sweet dishes, it can pretty much be sprinkled on everything else, says Hirsch.

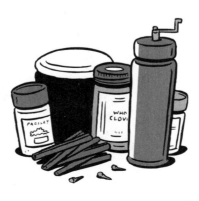

Make it hot. Paprika, red pepper and chili pepper are good flavor enhancers, Hirsch says. And they pack other health benefits. According to Dr. James Kenney, of the Pritikin Longevity Center, they may speed up your metabolism, helping you burn calories faster, and the intensity of the flavor may help curb your appetite so you eat less. Hot spices also offer a surprising—

and welcome—side effect: They can help prevent tooth decay by making your mouth water. But don't overdo the chili pepper. A study in Mexico suggests that in large amounts chili pepper may increase your risk of stomach cancer.

Capsaicin is a crystalline substance that makes a hot pepper hot. The higher the capsaicin content, the hotter the pepper. Paprika will color food as well as flavor it. Red pepper is often used in stews, baked beans and pickles. Chili pepper is milder and is a large ingredient of chili powder, which also usually contains garlic powder, oregano, cumin and salt. The powder is used on chili, barbecue, dips, potato chips, crackers, sauce and other Mexican food. Sweet pepper flakes are dehydrated bell peppers and can be used in Creole dishes, stews, soups and casseroles, according to Hirsch.

Use a pinch at a time. Keep these two things in mind: A pound of basil will season enough chicken cacciatore to feed 3,000 people, and a pound of oregano will flavor a pizza a day for a family of four for a year. You want to increase the amount of spices in low-salt recipes, but you don't want to overdo it, says Susan Massaron of the Pritikin Longevity Center. "If a recipe calls for one teaspoon of basil, some people put in a tablespoon to compensate for cutting the salt. Then the whole balance is out of whack," she says.

Experiment by adding a pinch and then tasting, adding a pinch and then tasting. If you're cutting out salt entirely, add about 25 percent more spice, she says.

Add early. Spicing food early allows the spices to better penetrate the food. When possible, double the marinating time of the food, recommends Hirsch. And save 25 percent of your seasonings to add during the last ten minutes of cooking.

Get in the Mix

We said experiment. But in case that word conjures up horrible memories of seventh-grade science class (Poor little Susie. Wonder if her eyebrows ever grew back?), we're going to let you cheat a little. Here are some common foods and, according to Rodale's Anita Hirsch, the spicy combinations that will make them taste tantalizing.

- **Poultry.** Rosemary and thyme; tarragon, marjoram, onion powder and garlic powder; cumin, bay leaf and saffron.
- **Seafood.** Cumin and oregano; tarragon, thyme, parsley flakes and garlic powder; thyme, fennel, saffron and red pepper.
- **Beef.** Thyme, bay leaf and minced onion; ginger, dry mustard and garlic powder; dill, onion and allspice; black pepper, bay leaf and cloves.
- **Pork.** Caraway, red pepper and paprika; thyme, dry mustard and sage; oregano and bay leaf; anise, ginger and sesame.
- **Potatoes.** Dill, onion powder, parsley flakes; caraway and onion powder; nutmeg and freeze-dried chives.
- **Rice.** Chili powder and cumin; curry powder, ginger and coriander; cinnamon, cardamom and cloves.
- **Pasta.** Basil, rosemary and parsley flakes; cumin, turmeric and red pepper; oregano and thyme.

Get fresh later. Dried herbs travel through a dish better than fresh ones, says Hirsch, so you'll want to use them when cooking. But, she says, fresh herbs are better to sprinkle on food just before serving.

Enjoy the daily grind. Keep a pepper mill filled with whole mustard near your range. A few grinds of mustard as you're cooking adds some zing to dishes, without an overpowering mustard flavor. Other spice seeds work as well, and you can even blend a few to your own taste.

Desserts

Halve Your Cake and Eat It Two

You can have the sweetest, saliva-inducing calorie-and-fat-laden-treat you can find. But you have to eat it the right way.

Take a bite. But don't swallow it. Hold it in your mouth. Let it slowly melt on your tongue. Enjoy it. Really taste it. Then have two more bites exactly the same way. That's it. You've eaten dessert. Save the rest for tomorrow.

"The first two or three bites are the best bites of anything. After that, you're trying to get back to the original bite. You're going on that memory," says nutrition consultant Diane Wilke. "I always tell people to pick whatever they want because it satisfies them more. Then, limit the portions.'"

There are two reasons to regularly eat dessert. First, when you deny yourself something you want, you generally end up stuffing yourself with much more of it than you normally would. Also, the dessert's sweetness is the signal to your brain that the meal is over. Without it, you may not feel full. And you'll be browsing through the kitchen all night looking for something to munch on.

Sometimes, healthy choices such as grapes, fruit-flavored yogurt or gingersnaps will turn off the brain. But sometimes it takes something really decadent.

If you're still craving decadence even after three bites, wait 15 minutes before taking a fourth. It takes a while for your brain to notice that you actually have eaten what it ordered. Chances are, after 15 minutes, the sweetness will have registered. And your craving will be gone.

Here are some other things to think about when eating dessert.

Sing sweetly. Try this trick: The next time you're drooling over some low-fat dessert in the grocery store aisle, start humming that obnoxious old Archies hit "Sugar Sugar." If it doesn't immediately kill whatever appetite you had, at least it will remind you to check the label to see if the manufacturer made up for the lack of fat by mixing in a ton of sugar. Look for low-fat cookies and other desserts with fruit juices added for sweetener, says Wilke.

Buyer beware. Some manufacturers cut out the fat by giving you a smaller product. A Hostess Low-Fat Cupcake has 50 fewer calories and 3.5 fewer grams of fat than the regular version. And it weighs 13 percent less. More compelling is the Twinkie story. A regular Twinkie's fat and calorie information is measured by using two cakes as a serving size. The low-fat Twinkie's information is measured by using one cake, so check the serving sizes. They may be comparing the fat content of 6 cookies versus 12 cookies, says Wilke.

Forgo false fruit. If a frozen fruit bar is what you crave, you might as well get some vitamins with your sugar. Look for fruit bars that supply at least 10 percent of the Daily Value for vitamin A or C. And on the ingredient list, make sure fruit or fruit puree is the first or second item.

Watch for stealth fat. Before you buy frozen yogurt or ice milk because you think it's healthier than ice cream, look at the label. Usually, frozen yogurt and ice milk have less fat than ice cream, but not always. A Kemps frozen yogurt bar has 17 grams of fat, compared to Häagen-Dazs's with 1 gram of fat. And FrozFruit Sweet 'n' Low Lower-Fat Ice Cream Bar has as much saturated fat—9 grams—as a Big Mac.

Go natural. You don't have to suffer with low-fat dryness. Some desserts are naturally low in fat, says Wilke, including gingersnaps, fig bars, graham crackers and angel food cake.

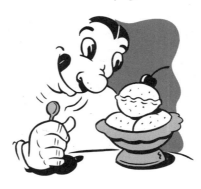

Part Three

Eating Out

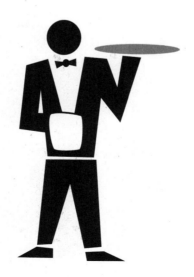

Restaurants

*You Can Always Get
What You Want*

> *If you're going to America, bring your
> own food.*
>
> —**Fran Lebowitz**

When you go to a restaurant, who's going to be in charge of what you eat?

How about the marketing guy who picked the colors in the glitzy sign out front and gave all the sandwiches movie-star names?

Or that waiter who's so happy to drive up the tab with another round of cocktails?

Or your poker buddy who thinks of chips and bean dip as an entrée?

No, no and no again. If you're an average American male, you dine out 4.3 times a week. That means you'd better take charge of what you eat in restaurants. Otherwise, a major portion of your food intake is sliding into your gullet unsupervised. Considering the truckloads of fat and calories gurgling onto restaurant serving dishes, you can't afford to surrender control every time you saunter into a dining hall.

"Twenty years ago, going to a restaurant really was a splurge, a special occasion. It probably didn't really matter what you ate," says Jayne Hurley, R.D., senior nutritionist at the Center for Science in the Public Interest in Washington, D.C., and a writer for the *Nutrition Action Health-letter.* "But now with 47 percent of the food dollar being spent outside of the home and a third of the calories being eaten outside of the home, it does matter.

What you put in your mouth in a restaurant counts."

Planning: Look before You Lunch

You hop into the car at lunchtime and wheel toward the main drag, where there are enough high-wattage fast-food signs to blind you even at midday. Let's see, where are we gonna eat . . . and before you know it, you're on a stool at the Greaseway Diner wolfing down cheeseburgers and onion rings.

Whoa. Back up. If you're going to eat right at restaurants, nutrition experts say, you need a plan before you hit the blacktop.

Be a leader—not a follower. Where you eat, of course, determines what you eat. So if you're traveling in a pack, be assertive and voice your preference of restaurants. Just in case you need to negotiate, have two or three alternatives already in mind—joints where you know they serve at least one meal to your nutritional specifications. In general, remember that homestyle American, French and continental restaurants lean toward rich and heavy dishes. Greek, Italian and Asian eateries are better bets.

Get one for the road. If you think you're likely to return to a restaurant, ask for a copy of the menu. Next time, decide what wholesome fare you're going to order before you even leave the house or office. That way, you won't be swayed by the devilish aroma of croissants or french fries before you've even gotten a table. When your mind is made up, your defenses are up.

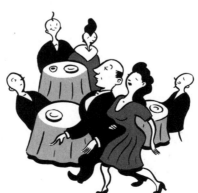

Go solo. Despite what The Eagles implied in their hit, "Already Gone," eating lunch all by yourself is not a bad thing. Psychologists theorize that you linger over your food, and eat more, when you have company. Georgia State University researchers found that when you eat with one companion, your consumption rises by 28 percent. With two companions, you eat 41 percent more, and with six or more dinner partners, you eat 76 percent more food.

Ordering: Grill the Waiter

Sometimes life just hangs in the balance. If you ask your waiter to slightly adjust the preparation of a meal, for instance, a crazed chef is liable to burst through the swinging doors and attack you with a meat cleaver. Right?

Not true at all, says Jonathan A. Zearfoss, a certified executive chef who teaches advanced cooking at The Culinary Institute of America in Hyde Park, New York. "Everybody has heard the stories—which are not true—about chefs who mistreat the food if someone asks for something out of the ordinary," Zearfoss says. "We emphasize here that one of the keys to success is being very attuned to what your customer wants. If it's not on the menu, a chef needs to be prepared to make it available."

Here are some reasonable matters to discuss with a waiter. Just make your requests without fanfare and without elaboration. Your cholesterol count is your business.

- What's the portion size? (Less than seven ounces of meat a day will do you.)
- Besides the main entrée, what else comes on the plate? (See if they'll give you a smaller hunk of meat and more vegetables and grains.)
- How is the food prepared? (Pan cooking means added fat. Grilled and roasted items tend to be lower in fat.)
- What kind of sauces are used? Can the sauces be served on the side? (Avoid

---

Terms of Endearment

When you see these cooking terms beside a menu item, you know you're on safer ground. They tend to keep calories and fat to a minimum.

Baked or roasted: Oven cooking, great for meat, fish and vegetables, like squash and potatoes.

Braised: Cooked in liquid.

Broiled or grilled: Cooked directly over or under the heat source and on a rack so the fat drains away.

Poached: Cooked quickly in liquid, often used for fish or boned poultry.

Sautéed or stir-fried: Quickly cooked in a pan or wok. Make sure it's done with minimal or no oil.

Steamed: Cooked in a container that exposes the food to steam. Adds no fat.

---

butter and cream.)
- Does a dish contain cheese or other products that would increase the fat content?
- Are substitutions possible? (Plain, steamed veggies rather than buttered; baked potato rather than fries; whole-grain bread rather than processed.)

Once you get your questions answered, here are some ideas for ordering up a nutritious meal.

Scout out the alternatives. Don't just pounce on the first menu item that jump-starts your saliva. Before you place an order, review the whole menu and identify all of the low-fat, high-carb options. Some restaurants highlight their heart-healthy fare with little symbols or feature such items in a special section of the menu.

Beware the "bargain." If a restaurant's special offer derails your nutritional efforts, that's no bargain at all. Avoid all-you-can-eat deals and "super-sizing" arrangements that encourage you to pack in more food than you had intended.

Get a little on the side. Salad dressings, on average, have 75 calories per tablespoon. By the time the kitchen staff has ladled it over your iceberg, you're way into the triple digits. Ask the waiter to serve dressing in a little container on the side so you can control the flow. Better yet, don't pour any dressing on your salad at all. Just dip your fork into the container, then stab at the salad—you'll still get the flavor, but only a fraction of the high-cal goop.

Eating: Divide and Conquer

Two elderly women are at a Catskills mountain resort and one of them says, "Boy, the food at this place is really terrible." The other one says, "Yeah, and such small portions."
—**Alvy in the movie Annie Hall**

If you're managing your meal correctly, small entrée portions actually work in your favor. Step one is to limit fat, which usually means limiting the size of the slab of meat that's often the centerpiece of your plate.

To compensate, order lots of whole grains, fruits and vegetables with your entrée, says Evelyn Tribole, R.D., a consulting nutritionist in Beverly Hills, California, and author of *Healthy Homestyle Cooking* and *Eating on the Run.*

If a restaurant won't downsize your entrée, take matters into your own hands. Trim your fat consumption by 50 percent with even the greasiest entrée imaginable by cutting the thing into two pieces and eating only half. If you tell the waiter to bag the other half right away, you'll remove the temptation to vacuum

Winners and Losers

Pop that menu open. Let's run down it and identify the reliable paths to healthy eating—and some of the roads best not taken.

Appetizers

Winners: Fruit, raw or steamed vegetables, tomato juice, dinner salad, seafood, vegetable or bean soup.

Losers: Fried vegetables, cream soups, pâté, fried cheese, tortilla chips.

Breads

Winners: Plain French bread, whole-grain bread, corn tortillas, flat bread, breadsticks, crackers.

Losers: Croissants, sweet rolls, muffins, biscuits, flour tortillas, fried breads, buttered anything.

Salads

Winners: Varied greens, dressing on the side, low-fat dressing, vinegar, a squeeze of lemon.

Losers: Standard dressing, egg yolks, olives, bacon bits, avocados, cheese.

down the whole entrée. Or just split it with a companion, which will shave a few bucks off the final tab.

Often you can order a more entertaining meal by ignoring the list of entrées altogether. "Appetizers are generally more interesting," says Zearfoss. "I can get three appetizers for the price of an entrée, so there's an economic factor. And appetizers tend to have more garnish than meat, so right there you're cutting back on the protein sources that would inevitably contain fat." Look for appetizers that are combined with salad, prepared with seafood or are smoked or cured meats.

Ethnic-based appetizers, like sushi,

Entrées

Winners: Seafood, pasta marinara, sushi, chicken teriyaki, chicken burritos, rice and chicken pilaf, shish kebab, lean meat (broiled, grilled or roasted).

Losers: Breaded, fried or sautéed meat, large slabs of meat, quiche, fried foods, potpies, heavy sauces or gravy.

Vegetables and Grains

Winners: Boiled, baked or steamed. Tomato sauces or herbed toppings.

Losers: Sautéed, fried, creamed or with added butter.

Desserts

Winners: Sorbets, ices, angel food cake, nonfat frozen yogurt.

Losers: Cheesecake, pie, ice cream, custards and pastries.

bruschetta or crostini with white bean puree, also are good choices. And beware of "family style" restaurants where appetizers tend to be heavily breaded and fried.

Here are other strategies to bring to the table in a restaurant.

Do drink the water. If you drink loads of water during your meal, you'll feel less hungry. Ask your waiter for a big glass and a bottle of mineral water or a pitcher of tap water.

Get souped up. To keep your consumption in check, ask for a soup appetizer. Researchers at Johns Hopkins University in Baltimore found that diners who began with tomato soup took in 25 percent fewer calories by the meal's end than people who started with cheese and crackers. The soup, they theorized, made diners feel fuller.

Jazz up the plate. Maybe the grilled chicken you ordered has the nutritious-but-bland syndrome. Ask the waiter for a little flavored vinegar, mustard or lemon juice to give that bird a kick.

When in Doubt, Go Fish

Feel the pressure mounting when you crack open a menu? At first, trying to put new nutritional knowledge into action when you're ordering can be mind-boggling. But even if you don't know your asparagus from a hole in the ground, there's a magic word that will instantly put your diet on firm footing. Tell your waiter: "Fish."

Fish is a wonderfully lean source of protein. Ounce-for-ounce, even the fattiest fish, like Atlantic salmon, has less than a third of the total fat you would get in a single serving of broiled rib-eye steak. Salmon, bluefish, trout, herring, mackerel, tuna and cod are also loaded with omega-3 fatty acids, which are thought to improve cholesterol levels and reduce the risk of heart disease.

Order your fish grilled, broiled, steamed, baked or blackened, says Hurley. Throw in a plain baked spud, an undressed salad (okay, okay, dash on some lemon or vinegar), a couple of rolls (no butter), and you have a meal that has half the fat of even the leanest Chinese or Italian dishes.

Avoid preparations that involve cheese, cream, butter or tartar sauce. And pass on fried seafood: Not only is it fatty but many restaurants fry with hydrogenated shortening that contains trans fats, which have been found to raise cholesterol levels, says Hurley.

Mediterranean Food

Order from the Heart

If Mediterranean cuisine is so hot, how come you don't see signs like "Joe's Mediterranean Restaurant" on every street corner? Well, *Mediterranean* actually covers an enormous variety of restaurants, cooking styles, ingredients and ethnic influences. (What do you want? There are at least 16 countries ringing the Mediterranean Sea.)

Scientists who declare the Mediterranean approach to be remarkably healthy are most interested in the regions where olive oil, a heart-healthy monounsaturate, is the main source of fat in the diet. You usually hear France, Italy, Spain and Greece discussed by way of example, because those countries have collected data on eating patterns among their people.

Scientists have suspected for decades that something healthy was going on in the Mediterranean region. The number one killer in America, heart disease, is rare in the Mediterranean. Same goes for a lot of other maladies, including diabetes, gallstones and high cholesterol. The people there have life spans longer than just about any other population, and the reason doesn't lie in educational level, wealth or health care spending, because the region tends to score low on those factors when compared to other industrialized countries.

The answers have become clearer. For one thing, people in the Mediterranean have historically followed an eating pattern much like the Food Guide Pyramid program in the United States—lots of beans, grains, fruits and vegetables, combined with a spare use of fats and sweets.

Despite all of the media attention that the Mediterranean approach has gained, it's hard to dismiss this near-vegetarian way of eating as another fad diet. It's actually a time-tested lifestyle reaching back thousands of years.

Eat Like a Mediterranean

Those omnipresent fresh fruits and vegetables in the Mediterranean diet play a number of roles in protecting the human body. For one thing, they're high in fiber. They're also rich in nutrients that help to lower cholesterol and blood pressure, as well as reduce the risk of heart disease and cancer. Among the protective substances are carotenoids and vitamins C and E.

Meat plays a minor role in Mediterranean meals. It's eaten only once or twice a week, and small amounts of chicken, pork or lamb are used more for flavor than bulk. And that's what keeps that population's consumption of heart-damaging saturated fat so low.

Because they have plenty of access to the sea, the Mediterraneans have plenty of fresh fish on their plates. That means they're getting loads of heart-healthy omega-3 fatty acids.

And boy do Mediterraneans go with the grain. When they're not ripping apart baguettes, they're forking down plates of pasta, polenta, couscous and other healthful grain foods. All of

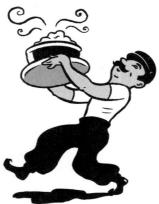

those complex carbohydrates translate into loads of low-fat energy.

The Right Fat

The way Mediterraneans eat, only 20 percent of the fat they consume is saturated—the heart-clogging stuff—compared to the 35 percent that the average American gets.

The dominant fat in Mediterranean cooking is olive oil. That's still fat, yes, but it's a monounsaturate—which lowers your serum cholesterol and therefore reduces your risk of heart disease and stroke. Besides, olive oil is high in vitamin E, which is thought to reduce the risk of cancer, heart disease and other serious maladies.

This is not to say that olive oil is a magic potion that you can use indiscriminately. "Although the Mediterranean populations do consume large quantities of olive oil and do have relatively low rates of heart disease, they differ from other populations in several respects other than just olive oil consumption," says Christopher Gardner, Ph.D., a research fellow at the Stanford Center for Research in Disease Prevention. "Some of the different characteristics of certain Mediterranean populations include different daily meal patterns, different types of food and alcoholic beverages, a midday siesta and much more daily physical activity. Olive oil and food items made with olive oil are a significant part of their diet, but it's really not fair to isolate that and say, 'Go ahead and consume all of the oil you want.'"

After all, olive oil *is* fat, which you want to consume in limited amounts. The wise eater, though, figures out how to reduce saturated fat (primarily from animal sources) and replace at least some of it with monounsaturates (like olive oil) or polyunsaturates (like corn oil). The result: A luscious eating style you can stick with, and a heart you can live with.

Ordering: Plain Speaking

So the next time you saunter into a Mediterranean bistro, all you need to do is tuck a napkin into your collar, snap your fingers and a heart-friendly platter of veggies and pasta will appear, right?

Not so fast, Zorba.

For advice on ordering, we appealed to Jacques Pépin, the renowned chef who grew up in the kitchen of his family's restaurant near Lyon, France. Unless you speak up, he says, a conventional restaurant meal can carry loads of hidden fat.

"Probably the biggest misunderstanding

Live Like a Mediterranean

As you may have gathered, the Mediterranean diet is not just a list of ingredients. It's a way of life.

Drink like a Frenchman. We're not talking about nightlife here, guys. What do the French do when they work up a thirst on a busy day? Cola? Juice? No, no, monsieur, far too many calories. More often than not, they pop open a bottle of water. And they have a big bread habit, too—tearing off big hunks of scrumptious stuff for a virtually fat-free complement to any meal.

Walk like a Spaniard. In many parts of the Mediterranean, walking is as much an ingrained lifestyle as driving is for Americans. In Italy they call it *passeggiata.* In Spain it's the *paseo.* They spend the evening strolling about the town center, visiting and talking. Beats channel-surfing any day.

Moderate like an Italian. In Italy pizzas do not come in Sistine Chapel proportions. They're no bigger than a dinner plate, contain far less cheese than Americans use and are simply sprinkled with tomato, basil and oil. And an Italian dessert is commonly fruit. Shoveling a bowlful of ice cream out of a bucket from the home freezer is unheard of. You have to go out for it, and it's served in small, expensive cones.

is pasta and salad," Pépin says. "I mean, there is nothing wrong with pasta or salad, but in a restaurant you are going to have a green salad with approximately three tablespoons of olive oil—it's already close to 500 calories. Then you want a pasta and say, 'I don't want any sauce on it.' But the amount of oil, butter and cheese incorporated into that pasta can still amount to 1,500 calories.

"Because you just had a plain pasta without any sauce and a green salad, you feel very righteous, so you have two pieces of chocolate cake. So you come out of there with over 3,000 calories and say, 'Well, I had a very light lunch—I just had a green salad and pasta.'"

For the salad, Pépin says, tell the waiter you want the dressing on the side so you can control the amount of oil. For that "plain" pasta, be very specific. "You could say, 'Give me a little bit of grated Parmesan cheese, and I just want a tablespoon of olive oil in it, and I don't want anything else. So be sure to tell the chef. Or if you don't want to do it, just bring the pasta to me hot and plain with a bit of oil—I'll put it on myself.'"

Passionate about Pasta

Back when you were no taller than a doorknob, you called pasta "sketti" and the weight-conscious legions wouldn't go near the stuff. *Mama mia,* how things change.

"Italian is real simple. The secret is the pasta," says Jayne Hurley of the Center for Science in the Public Interest. "As long as you get a plate of spaghetti or linguine, you can top it with tomato sauce, marinara sauce, red or white clam sauce, meat sauce, even meatballs, and you're practically guaranteed a lower-fat meal."

Hurley and her co-workers bought 15 popular dishes from 21 midpriced Italian restaurants across the United States and shipped the food to a lab to be analyzed for caloric and fat content. "There's a lot of misinformation out

there about what's good and what's bad," she says. "Spaghetti and meatballs was usually not on anybody's recommended list if you were looking at the restaurant books written prior to our analysis. It actually came out to be one of the lower-fat choices."

Here are other things you'll want to know about dining in Italian restaurants.

Pan the lasagna. Sure, it has those big, wide noodles in it, but lasagna is really a meat-and-cheese dish (read: high-fat) with a little pasta tossed in. "Unfortunately, lasagna is the most popular dish ordered at Italian restaurants," Hurley says. "But a typical order of lasagna is like eating two Big Macs."

Beware the bread. You always knew garlic bread was potent stuff. But the problem isn't getting dragon breath. It's that garlic bread is typically sopping with oil or butter. Instead, order plain Italian bread and, if you must, knife a thin smear of butter onto it.

Avoid Alfredo. The *Nutrition Action Healthletter* folks dubbed fettuccine Alfredo "heart attack on a plate." Why? How's 97 grams of fat per serving sound?

"I've been a nutritionist for 15 years and I have never seen anything this bad," says Hurley. "Two-and-a-half-days' worth of saturated fat. It's really nice and naive to tell people there's no such thing as good or bad foods, only good or bad diets, and as long as you eat carefully the rest of the day, you can fit this food into your diet. *Wrong.* You have to be willing to eat nothing but fruits and vegetables for two and a half days if you want to 'fit' fettuccine Alfredo into a healthy diet."

Any way you slice it. Ordering a nutritious pizza is easy as pie. Just use a little restraint.

From the crust you get carbs, from the cheese you get protein and calcium and from the sauce and vegetable toppings you get vitamins A and C. Most pizzas get a respectable 25 to 30 percent of their calories from fat. But be careful: Add a meat topping and the fat count jumps above 40 percent.

Mexican Food

You Can Lean to Lighter Fare

If you want healthy Mexican food, you should *really* head for the border sometime. When U.S. restaurants adapt Mexican cuisine, they often make major mistakes, like tossing in buckets and buckets of cheese, sour cream and oil, which are barely present in the original food.

Mexicans actually tend to dine on high-carbohydrate, low-fat fare. Corn is a staple of the true Mexican diet, particularly in the form of tortillas made from cornmeal and water—no oil. Warm a tortilla on the griddle, layer on some beans, salsa and a little shredded meat and you have an authentic south-of-the-border meal. To tickle the taste buds, there are marinades and salsas made from chilies, other spices, garlic, onion, water and little, if any, oil. Lean and luscious, amigo.

Most of the Mexican food issuing from U.S. kitchens is a different story. The *Nutrition Action Healthletter* staff analyzed 15 popular dishes at 19 midpriced Mexican restaurants. Only one entrée, chicken fajitas, got less than 30 percent of its calories from fat. Most of the meals, with the help of "platter" servings of refried beans, sour cream and guacamole, provided an entire day's worth of fat in one sitting.

The good news is that some Mexican restaurants are making it easier to protect your arteries. Two of the country's largest table-service Mexican restaurant chains have overhauled their menus. Chi-Chi's and El Torito stripped some fat out of existing dishes and also invented new, lower-fat items. "They put fat information on the menu to guide

people, and they started offering nonfat sour cream, reduced-fat cheese and refried beans that were made without oil," says Jayne Hurley of the Center for Science in the Public Interest.

And Taco Bell posts an eight-item, reduced-fat "Border Lights" menu. The Light Soft Taco Supreme, for instance, has 5 grams of fat while the original has 15. "They used leaner ground beef. They used reduced-fat cheese and nonfat sour cream. They cut back on the oil in their beans. And—*voila*—there's this fabulous menu that's one of the most groundbreaking things I've witnessed in the fast-food world," says Hurley.

Other forward-thinking restaurants are offering such items as brown rice, whole-wheat bread, nonfat black beans, lower-fat cheese, marinated or steamed vegetables and a sour-cream-and-yogurt blend as a condiment.

Tortilla Fats

Your first challenge in a Mexican restaurant usually comes uninvited: that complimentary basket of aromatic, toasty tortilla chips fried in enough oil to make OPEC jealous. A basket of 50 chips carries two-thirds of your fat allotment for the day. But if you're not careful, they'll evaporate before you can crack the menu.

"The problem with the chips is unconscious eating—eating amnesia," says nutritionist Evelyn Tribole. "You fill up on the chips and then your dinner comes and you are eating on top of that— you are overeating."

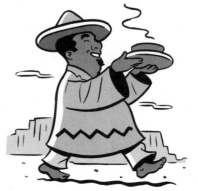

To limit your chip consumption, Tribole suggests, decide up front how many you will eat. Remove that number from the basket and place them on your plate. When those are gone, you're done—no double-dipping.

Alternatives: Tell the waiter to take all of the chips

In Search of Sensational Salsa (and Chips)

For years they trained, reaching precariously across the buffet table at parties. Prowling Mexican restaurants. Late night brush-up sessions in front of the television. Finally, our 12 taste-testers were ready. Their mission: Take five brands of heart-healthy tortilla chips and five brands of chunky, medium-spice salsa. Rate them on a scale of 1 to 10, with 10 being the highest. And let the chips fall where they may. The results:

The Salsas

Pace Thick and Chunky Salsa

Per serving: **10 calories, no fat**
Score: **7.2**
Comment: **"Full and chunky. Satisfying. Hotter than other mediums."**

Old El Paso Homestyle Chunky Salsa

Per serving: **5 calories, no fat**
Score: **6.1**
Comment: **"Tangy, but not hot. Looks homemade, with lots of veggie chunks."**

Chi-Chi's Chunky Restaurant Salsa

Per serving: **10 calories, no fat**
Score: **5.2**
Comment: **"Somewhat watery. Fairly spicy taste. Good blend of jalapeño peppers and tomato."**

Ortega Thick and Chunky Salsa

Per serving: **10 calories, no fat**
Score: **4.4**
Comment: **"I was looking for salsa, not an onion dip."**

Herr's Chunky Salsa

Per serving: **12 calories, no fat**
Score: **4.2**
Comment: **"More like tomato sauce than salsa."**

The Tortilla Chips

Original Smart Temptations Tortilla Chips

Per serving: **110 calories, 1 gram of fat**
Score: **7.4**
Comment: **"Excellent. Fresh, crunchy, a bit salty. The only plain chip I would eat by itself."**

Baked Tostitos (low fat)

Per serving: **110 calories, 1 gram of fat**
Score: **6.8**
Comment: **"Good tortilla taste—crisp, zesty, a little crumbly. Generous size."**

Barbara's Bakery Tortilla Chips (white corn)

Per serving: **120 calories, 4 grams of fat**
Score: **6.4**
Comment: **"Good, full, zesty taste."**

Note: This "reduced-fat" chip was the only one with more than 1 gram of fat per serving. We could only find it in ranch flavor, while the others were au naturel.

Guiltless Gourmet Baked Tortilla Chips (white corn)

Per serving: **110 calories, 1 gram of fat**
Score: **5.3**
Comment: **"Crispy. A bit bland."**

Bearitos Organic Baked Tortilla Chips (yellow corn)

Per serving: **110 calories, 1 gram of fat**
Score: **3.4**
Comment: **"Tasted like paper."**

away immediately, says Hurley. Another idea: Ask to have the chips served with the meal, suggests Tribole. Or ask the waiter if he has any baked tortilla chips, the kind commonly available in grocery stores. Or ask him for soft tortillas, which you can dip into the salsa, says Tribole.

Do You Know Beans about Ordering?

You'll find a number of terms on a Mexican restaurant menu that translate pretty much the same: high fat. These warning flags, says Antonio M. Gotto, Jr., M.D., Ph.D., chairman of the Department of Medicine at Baylor College of Medicine in Houston and co-author with Lynne W. Scott, R.D., of *The Living Heart Guide to Eating Out*, include:

- Carnitas: Fried beef or pork.
- Chorizo: Spicy pork sausage.
- Quesadillas: Tortillas filled with meat and cheese, then fried.
- Refried beans: Mashed beans cooked with fat.

Here are other things to consider while ordering in a Mexican restaurant.

Sidestep those traps. If you can, order à la carte, which means you'll get the bare-bones item named on the menu without all of the trimmings that conspire to stop your heart. If fatty ingredients, like sour cream, cheese and guacamole, come with the meal anyway, request that they be served on the side, where you can control the amount you eat, says Tribole. You can add as much salsa or pico de gallo as you like—they are nonfat, adds Hurley.

Skip the rice and beans. It seems almost heretical, but in most Mexican restaurants, you're better off *not* ordering rice and beans. Why? The folks at the Center for Science in the Public Interest found that a ¾-cup serving of rice at a typical Mexican restaurant packs about a third of your daily maximum of sodium. The beans have almost as much.

And to make matters worse, a ¾-cup serving of refried beans is loaded with a third of your daily maximum of saturated fat.

The bottom line. If you just ate the side orders—rice and beans, sour cream and guacamole—without any main entrée, you'd still get almost two-thirds of a day's total fat, and three-quarters of a day's saturated fat and sodium.

Toss the menu. Ask your waiter if the chef offers any off-the-menu items, like grilled fish or chicken breast, suggests Dr. Gotto.

Always cast your vote. Don't hesitate to make a special request of your waiter, even if you doubt he'll be able to deliver. Think of each request as another vote for healthy food. "It's always worth asking, because it's up to the consumer," says Hurley. "If enough people ask, then restaurants will actually start carrying this stuff." As they say in Chicago, "Vote early, and vote often."

Fajitas: It's a Wrap

Now that you know how to order, here's what to order. Your best bet: fajitas, which are usually strips of marinated meat sautéed with onions and green peppers, wrapped up in a soft tortilla. For extra kick, layer on some salsa.

"You can get shrimp, vegetable or chicken—as long as you skip the sour cream, guacamole and refried beans, which are loaded with fat and typically come with the fajitas," Hurley says. "The best bet is to find out if you can get some nonfat sour cream and beans made without oil."

Other fairly safe territory suggested by Hurley and Tribole:

- Appetizers: black bean soup, seviche (marinated fish), gazpacho (spicy, cold soup), tortilla soup
- Entrées: soft chicken taco, chicken burrito, chicken and rice, whole beans and rice
- Dessert: flan, fruit, fruit ices

Some dishes to avoid: chile relleno, cheese enchilada, chimichanga, nachos, deep-fried churros (doughnuts), ground beef and pork in any dish.

Asian Food

To Eat Well, Bow to Tradition

Ah, the mysteries of the Orient.
- Japanese-American men have three to four times more heart disease than their counterparts living in Japan, according to a Honolulu Heart Program study done by the National Heart, Lung and Blood Institute.
- Chinese-American men have four to seven times more colorectal cancer than men in China, according to a Stanford University School of Medicine study.

Why are Asian men in the United States more vulnerable to killer diseases? They've strayed from the ultra-low-fat diets of their ancestors. They're eating American.

When they eat in the traditional style, Chinese people get three times the fiber that a typical American consumes. They also take in half the fat and have half the cholesterol levels.

Eureka! The answer to America's health problems has just struck you: Convert all of our steak-and-burger houses into Chinese restaurants!

Nice try. But the food you're served in a North American Chinese restaurant isn't the same stuff that's keeping people trim and healthy on the other side of the Pacific Ocean. In China, people typically eat as much as six cups of rice at a sitting, a generous amount of vegetables and a few shreds of meat.

Americanized Chinese food gets the emphasis backward: little rice, mounds of meat, deep-fried appetizers and pools of sodium-charged soy sauce. "My rule of thumb is this: Every cup of entrée should be accompanied by a cup of steamed rice," says Jayne Hurley of the Center for Science in the Public Interest.

Ordering: Go Steam-Powered

Many Chinese restaurants are sensitive to the demand for more healthful food and provide detailed descriptions on their menus. If there's not enough information for you to judge a dish by, ask your waiter what's in it and how it's fixed. If the dish is not quite what you hoped for, most restaurants are glad to tailor food to your specifications.

For instance, to keep the salt level down in stir-fry, ask the waiter to use low-sodium soy sauce. If you're ordering chow mein, ask for steamed vegetables instead of those greasy fried noodles. To curb fat in an Indian restaurant, have that curry sauce served on the side.

Here are more tips for giving your Asian food a nutritious tweak when you're ordering, says Hurley. The advice here, by the way, is not for Chinese restaurants only. Many of these techniques work for Japanese, Vietnamese, Thai and Indian, too.

Get steamed. Steaming, of course, is a no-oil cooking method, so it's a choice that goes straight to the heart. It also leaves you with a wide range of delectable Chinese dishes to choose from. For appetizers order steamed dumplings instead of fried egg rolls. Make sure you're getting steamed rice with your entrée, not fried rice. If a meat-heavy dish has caught your eye, go ahead and order it. But ask for an order of steamed vegetables, too, and add it to your entrée.

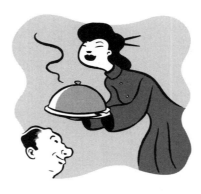

Even if you can't find it on the menu, ask your waiter for steamed vegetables with chicken or shrimp. From a nutrition standpoint, it's one of your best bets, and just about any

Chinese chef will know how to do a top-notch job of it. With light-meat chicken this dish would be only about 175 calories, with five grams of fat. Shrimp, even leaner: 22 calories and a quarter-gram of fat.

Eschew cashews. Nuts are fat pills. One large, oil-roasted cashew carries about a gram of fat. Imagine how that adds up when you pour a half-cup of them into an entrée. So tell your waiter to hold the nuts. For some low-fat crunch in your lunch try water chestnuts instead. Or, if your kung pao chicken just wouldn't have enough "pow" without those peanuts, tell the waiter two or three tablespoons max.

Read 'em and weep. When you open the menu, watch out for these terms.

- Crispy or fried. Translation: dunked in fat.
- Sweet and sour. Translation: The meat was first deep-fried, then stir-fried with the vegetables, adding even more oil.

Sorting through the Dishes

As with any cuisine, some Chinese dishes are secretive fat reservoirs and others are refreshingly lean. To defend yourself, study up in advance.

When the *Nutrition Action Healthletter* analyzed 15 common Chinese dishes, these got the best ratings.

- Szechuan shrimp (stir-fried in hot sauce) (four cups): 927 calories, 18 percent calories from fat, 19 grams of fat, 2,457 milligrams of sodium
- Stir-fried vegetables (four cups): 746 calories, 22 percent calories from fat, 19 grams of fat, 2,153 milligrams of sodium
- Shrimp with garlic sauce (three cups): 945

calories, 25 percent calories from fat, 27 grams of fat, 2,951 milligrams of sodium

And these were rated the worst.

- Egg roll (one): 190 calories, 52 percent calories from fat, 11 grams of fat, 463 milligrams of sodium
- Moo shu pork (four cups): 1,228 calories, 47 percent calories from fat, 64 grams of fat, 2,593 milligrams of sodium
- Kung pao chicken (five cups): 1,620 calories, 42 percent calories from fat, 76 grams of fat, 2,608 milligrams of sodium

Chopsticks: Picking It Up

You don't want to look like a rube when the boss takes you out for Chinese food. That's one reason for learning to use chopsticks.

But chopsticks encourage healthy eating, too. When you use a set of twigs to lift your food out of the serving tray and onto your rice, a lot of that fatty sauce drains away. Try to leave behind any excess egg and nuts, too. Chopsticks also force your eating into a leisurely pace, making it less likely that you'll gorge yourself—an old health spa trick.

So here's how to use chopsticks.

- Lay one chopstick in the crook between your thumb and forefinger, and let it rest against the tip of the ring finger of the same hand. This bottom chopstick doesn't move when you pick up food.
- Now, lay in the top chopstick, holding it the way you would a dart—between the thumb and first two fingers. This is the chopstick that does all of the moving.
- Tap the chopsticks on the tabletop to get the ends even with each other.
- Open and close the tips. You've created a little puppet mouth that can pick up even the tiniest grain of rice.

Steak and Barbecue

Time to Beef Up Your Defenses

Sure, you eat a healthy meal at a restaurant like Ted's Tofu Temptations. Ask for red meat there and you get a slice of beefsteak tomato. You saunter out smiling and smug with your masterful knowledge of how to feed the human body.

But for a real test of your nutritional fortitude, check out the fatfest at your local steak house or barbecue joint. Slabs of beef large enough to earn their own zip code. Baked spuds with moon-size dollops of butter. Racks of ribs resembling a barbecued xylophone. You're in the lion's den now, Daniel.

"I don't want to say don't eat those things. Steak in particular is a great source of zinc and other trace minerals. It's an excellent source of protein," says Liz Applegate, Ph.D., nutrition editor for *Runner's World* magazine. "So it's an item that can be had in the diet. The motto here is moderation.

"Steak houses are known for huge, huge servings. What guy is going to push away a plate of ribs? Or push away a ten-ounce steak? This is the tough part. Just tell yourself you're really getting on the average two to three times—if not four to five times—the amount of protein you should be getting."

It's the Size That Counts

Here are defensive measures you can take to ensure you have a good time at a steak house without suffering a fat overdose.

Think small. Forget that megaslab of steak touted at the top of the menu. "There is nothing wrong with having a steak, but order the smaller size. Believe me, that is still bigger than you can imagine," says nutritionist Evelyn Tribole. "The general rule of thumb is that you don't need more than six or seven ounces of meat in a day. A serving of meat the size of a deck of cards is about three ounces."

Share the wealth. Can't find a three- or four-ounce steak on the menu? Well, split a larger one with a friend, or slide half into a doggie bag, and then load up your plate with low-fat items, like vegetables and fruit. "Share with somebody and then say, 'I'm going to get a salad. I'm going to get a baked potato.' Put other items on the plate. Crowd out the steak or the ribs," says Dr. Applegate.

Check the options. Scan the menu. Maybe the restaurant offers meals that use beef as an ingredient rather than as a single discus on the plate. Shish kebab, stew, stir-fry and chili, for example, increase your vegetable intake and save you from that gee-I-got-a-puny-steak feeling.

Know your meat. To cut down on fat while eating out, stick with sirloin steaks or those from the tenderloin, such as filet mignon, suggests Anita Hirsch, R.D., a nutritionist at the Rodale Food Center in Emmaus, Pennsylvania. Avoid anything with rib in the name, such as prime rib, rib eye or spareribs, because they  contain more fat. To reduce the fat even more, be sure to trim off all the visible fat. Ask about cooking methods. Broiling and braising will be the lowest in fat. Poultry, of course, is generally lower in fat than red meat, and chicken breast is lower in saturated fat and cholesterol than legs or wings—especially Buffalo wings. To reduce fat even more, don't eat the poultry skin.

A Gentle Ribbing

If you want to start a bar fight, you needn't dally with politics or religious talk. Just profess, loudly, to know the one true meaning of barbecue.

In Georgia it's a vinegar-ketchup-mustard sauce. North Carolina barbecue is slow-smoked, shredded pork in vinegar sauce. In Kentucky they barbecue mutton. New Englanders grill lobster, hard-shell clams and mackerel. In the northwestern states it's salmon grilled over alder wood. In Texas it's slow-cooked beef brisket, while they barbecue just about anything that moves in Kansas City—though spareribs are a favorite. And in California, someone will serve you grilled eggplant if you're not careful.

Problem is, barbecue to a lot of people means one of the fattiest parts of the pig or cow—the ribs.

"Ribs? I have nothing positive to say about ribs," says Dr. Applegate. "But they taste good to a lot of people, and I don't like to say, 'Oh, you shouldn't eat those—they're bad.' To me, there's no such thing as a bad food. It's really how much you eat of it. So your best bet is to go in with people, share, talk a lot, drink a beer or two—you know, fill yourself up with something other than just this humongous serving of ribs."

Barbecued chicken is a lower-fat alternative, Tribole says. To make it even more healthful, peel the skin off before you eat. If you lose all of the seasoning in the process, ask for a little container of the barbecue sauce and dip the meat into it. The sauce is fine—all the fat is in the skin.

And finally, fellows, remember that immaturity and eating are a dangerous combination. Recite ribald limericks if you must or hang spoons from your nose, but do not in-dulge in a rib-eating contest.

"It just doesn't pay off," says Dr. Applegate. "I mean, no offense to men, but there's some kind of test of manhood—who can eat more. Even if you win the competition, you lose in the long run, because you're just loaded down with three days' worth of fat. You're overloaded with protein. It's going to have to be dealt with by the body, and it's just not wise."

A Saucy Selection

Now you can stay home and get "sauced."

We're not talking Watney's Red Barrel or Jack Daniel's sour mash here. We mean King Street Blues and Sonny Bryan's Smokehouse and Mark's Feed Store.

They're all famous barbecue joints. Forget that road trip you were going to take, ribbing it from (respectively) Alexandria, Virginia, to Dallas, Texas, to Middletown, Kentucky. Call the mail-order company Specialty Sauces at 1-800-728-2371 (1-800-SAUCES1) and they'll ship you a box of tried-and-true sauces that are in use at the nation's favorite barbecue stands. They also stock hot sauces and salsas.

"We're very much into the gourmet end of it," says company president Aaron Krumbein. "We think it's very cool to have a selection of sauces that come from every region of the country. So when you get a barbecue sauce from Texas, it's most definitely different from something you get from the Midwest. Midwestern sauces are redder and sweeter and Texas sauces are more brown and smoky. The sauces from states such as Tennessee and Georgia are milder and less full-bodied, but the people there will tell you that theirs is real barbecue."

Is there a region that wouldn't?

"No, of course not."

Fast Food

You Deserve a Break Today

I don't suppose you have a chili dog. I'd even eat it raw.
—Scott Glenn, invited to dine on sashimi and sake in the movie The Challenge

In 1948 brother restaurateurs Mac and Dick McDonald got an all-American idea. Why not apply mass-production concepts to a hamburger stand? Narrow the menu. Decide in advance what condiments the customer will get. Use throwaway packaging. Eliminate waiters, busboys and dishwashers to cut operating costs in half. The customer benefits, too: fast service and 15-cent burgers.

An entrepreneurial milk shake machine salesman named Ray Kroc loved the idea and started selling McDonald's franchises. Several years later Kroc bought the whole company. And within a few decades Americans were scarfing fast-food burgers at the rate of 200 per second.

As the bottom line grew for fast-food chains, so did bottoms and waistlines. Fat consumption in the United States has risen 31 percent in the last 75 years. While many items in fast-food restaurants get half their calories from fat, nudging Americans toward cardiovascular disease, that's not the only problem worrying nutrition scientists. A heavy reliance on the limited menus in fast-food restaurants makes it less likely that you'll eat a variety of foods—leading to nutritional deficiencies.

"It's important to note that eating like this is more the norm than eating at home, sitting at your dinner table," says Dr. Liz Applegate of *Runner's*

World magazine. "It's just more common that people eat out, particularly for men, since they're less apt to prepare their food."

Telling you to swear off fast-food stands, of course, would be like telling the Colorado River to reverse direction. The truth is, you don't have to perform unnatural acts in order to eat well. Just remember some guidelines whenever you get a hankering for quick cuisine.

Map Out the Territory

First, do some homework.

"It's worth it, for one week, just to go to your different fast-food places and say, 'May I have some nutritional information?'" says Dr. Applegate. "They'll hand you a booklet. Stick it in the bathroom by the toilet or something and read through it. Become familiar with your stomping grounds as far as fast-food outlets."

Every once in a while, ask for a new brochure and recheck your favorite menu items. Fast-food companies frequently tinker with their products, and you could easily find, for instance, that the chicken sandwich you've been ordering is suddenly using a full-fat mayonnaise dressing instead of the low-fat spread that once caught your eye.

Here are more tips that will steer you in a nutritious direction.

Have a plan, man. "Before you get within 20 feet of the smell of a fast-food outlet,

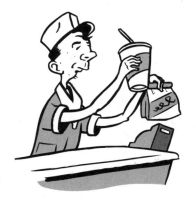

you need to say, 'When I walk in, I'm going to get . . .' Otherwise you get overtaken by the smell and the pictures. When you walk in and are indecisive, you sit down with more food than you should be eating," Dr. Applegate warns.

Forgo fried foods. Fish and chicken may sound healthy, but frying them can drench them in so much fat that they rival a hamburger. Stick with the broiled or roasted sandwiches.

Bigger isn't better. Forget those megameals that cost just a few dimes extra. "Stay away from anything called jumbo, giant, supersized or colossal," says Jayne Hurley of the Center for Science in the Public Interest. "That's generally a dead give-away that something's loaded with calories and fat."

Entrées: A Quick Course in Nutrition

Ironically, the starring attractions at many burger joints never had "moo" in their vocabulary. When *Prevention* magazine named the ten most reasonable fast-food sand-wiches—judging by fat, sodium and palatability—half of them were chicken. Even some of the chicken sandwiches need a little help. At Burger King, for example, tell them to hold the fatty sauce and you'll have a meal worth clucking about.

Here are other ways to ride herd on the beef.

Lean toward the lean. The occasional hamburger is not going to hurt you. When you order one, though, remember that they're not all created equal. "The best bet is the McLean Deluxe burger, which is the only lean hamburger available," Hurley says. "If you're not at McDonald's, then the best bet is probably a small burger. The reason that it's lower in fat is simply because you're not getting much meat."

Pile on the tomato. Not many men get excited about a lone puck of beef slapped onto a bun. To dress it up, ask for lettuce and tomato (for a nutrient boost, ask for extra slices). Add some mustard or ketchup, if you like, but draw the line at special sauces, mayon-naise and cheese, all of which can add globs of

---

> ## Boys and Grills: The Quiz
>
> Sink your teeth into these burger brainteasers (or is it greasers?), then turn the page to find the answers.
>
> 1. What's the full name of the mooching muncher in the Popeye cartoons? ("I'd gladly pay you Tuesday for a hamburger today.")
> 2. Name three movies with all of these elements: fast food, college student angst and a title that directly addresses the subject at hand—fast food.
> 3. Name three pop/rock songs with "burger" in the title.
> 4. On a typical day what percentage of the American population eats in a fast-food restau-rant? (a) 7 percent, (b) 15 percent, (c) 20 per-cent, (d) 28 percent or (e) 35 percent.
> 5. Who was the first person to portray that clown of ground round, Ronald McDonald?

---

fat. If you must have sauce, get some on the side so that you can control the amount you consume, says Hurley.

Think ethnic. Next time you get a case of burgerlust, consider the ethnic alternatives that still deliver fast-food convenience. At Mex-ican restaurants bean-and-soft-tortilla combos are a good bet. At Chinese restaurants it's easy to find a quick vegetarian dish (ask for loads of steamed rice), suggests Dr. Applegate. Or order up a slice or two of pizza—but stick with plain cheese or a vegetable topping. Skip the olives and meat, and pass on the greasy deep-dish variety.

Side Issues: Salad Strategy

Think of side orders as little nutritional torpedoes lurking in your fast-food restaurant. Hash browns? Twelve grams of fat—more than a regular hamburger. Apple pie? Even worse.

Large order of fries? It has about the same amount of fat and calories as a Quarter Pounder.

"French fries are one of the most common things people get with a sandwich," Hurley says. "But getting a supersize order of french fries is like eating a Big Mac. People think of french fries as a side dish. They're really not. It's like eating another whole sandwich. I usually tell people to get two grilled chicken sandwiches if one isn't enough, rather than getting the fries. Or get a salad."

Ah, salad. A plate full of vegetables in a little plastic carton—hard to mess up. Just rip open one of those squishy packets of dressing and squirt it on, right? Well, first look at the fine print on that packet.

"A salad with regular dressing can put you in Big Mac territory, so get the reduced-calorie or light dressing," Hurley advises.

Some of those packets contain two servings of dressing and that means a couple hundred calories. (Was somebody planning for a banquet?) Those packets also can be mini salt mines, some providing more than 1,100 milligrams of sodium—nearly half a day's worth. Others score more respectably in the 200s.

It also helps to use your head. The word "salad" is not a magic wand that will convert fatty foods into lean. So when you pile meat, cheese and sour cream into a fried taco shell with a bed of lettuce, you nearly max out your day's allotment of fat and get a 1,100 milligram jolt of sodium at the same time.

To quench your thirst, tank up on orange juice, 1 percent milk or water. Diet soda and coffee also will keep the calorie count down, says Hurley. McDonald's is known for its reasonably trim shakes: 340 calories and five grams of fat for a small vanilla, chocolate or strawberry shake.

Breakfast: Off to a Good Start

It's a shame to start your day with a nutritional strike against you, but it's so easy to do in a fast-food restaurant. A sausage-and-egg biscuit, for example, will typically load you up with 520 calories, 35 grams of fat, 1,200 milligrams of sodium and 275 milligrams of cholesterol.

Yes, you deserve a break from all that. Here's how to break in the new day without breaking training.

Go with the grain. Some of the most popular fast-food stands offer cereal. Try one of the nonsugary brands, like Cheerios or Wheaties, and splash on some low-fat milk. You'll have a good start for the day on calcium and vitamins A and C.

Stack 'em up. An order of pancakes with syrup is one of your best bets in a fast-food restaurant. Be sure to pass on the butter, though, and avoid platters that include bacon or sausage. Also, forget the French toast—it's usually deep-fried.

Don't get sideswiped. Sure, those hotcakes look lonely, but don't crowd the plate with heart-clogging extras, like bacon or hash browns. Look for high-carbohydrate add-ons, like a nonfat bran muffin and orange juice.

Sneak it in. Maybe the most convenient stop on your way to work has a pitiful range of nutritious items. So take matters into your own hands: Cart in a piece of fruit or one of those miniboxes of cereal, says Dr. Applegate. Then order just the good stuff when you get to the restaurant—hotcakes and low-fat milk, for instance.

Get jammin'. Use as little butter and margarine as possible. Jam will dress up your toast or English muffin with fewer calories and no fat.

Make it really fast. One of the main appeals of fast food is that it's, well, fast. So if you're really in a hurry, try this: Order low-fat milk, fruit juice and an unbuttered English muffin. You'll be on your way in no time, but with a complete breakfast in your stomach.

Ham it up. If you love those handy breakfast sandwiches, and absolutely must have meat on them, order one with ham or Canadian bacon instead of sausage or regular bacon.

Will That Sub Sink Your Diet?

With all of the lean and low-salt deli meats, cheeses and condiments on the market, the ultimate fast-food solution seems obvious: sandwich and sub shops! Nice try, but you still can't dive in with eyes closed and mouth open.

When the *Nutrition Action Healthletter* folks tested 175 sandwiches from shops across the country, they discovered "a minefield of fat and salt."

Here are some things Jayne Hurley and the staff at the Center for Science in the Public Interest recommend to keep in mind.

Hold the mayo. Delis seem to get mayonnaise delivered by tanker truck. Unless you speak up, expect them to trowel it onto your sandwich. Just a tablespoon can triple the fat content of a turkey breast sandwich.

Dress it right. Nutritious does not have to mean tasteless. Get lettuce, tomato and onions on your sandwich for plenty of delicious snap, squish and crunch. For a creamy touch ask for light cheese and low-fat dressing, and get whole-wheat bread.

Alter the lineup. You already know that bacon, lettuce and tomato sandwiches aren't steamed broccoli. But did you know they have more sodium, fat and calories than any burger you can buy at McDonald's? If you just have to have one, ask for lower-fat turkey bacon instead of regular. Or at least pluck out half the bacon before you bite down.

Make sure meat-free is also fat-free. Before you order a vegetarian sandwich, ask what's in it. Sprouts, onion, cucumber, lettuce and tomato? Fine. Avocado, cheese and mayo dressing? Fat.

Boys and Grills: The Answers

If you're just browsing, turn back a page to find the "Boys and Grills" quiz. No fair peeking at the answers below.

1. The burger moocher: J. Wellington Wimpy.

2. Here are our selections for slider cinema.

- *Fast Food* (1989): Two college party animals open a burger joint and use an aphrodisiac in their "secret sauce."

- *Hamburger . . . The Motion Picture* (1986): With his inheritance hinging on whether he gets a college diploma, a young man enters Burgerbuster University to get a degree in fast-food management.

- *Diner* (1982): College students wrestle with growing up in 1950s Baltimore.

No score for the war movie *Hamburger Hill*, and shame on you for trying to slip that past us.

3. Songs to hum the next time you stroll through the golden arches: "Burgers and Fries" by Charley Pride, "Cheeseburger in Paradise" by Jimmy Buffett and "Hot Dogs and Hamburgers" by John Mellencamp.

Two points for "Two Triple Cheese, Side Order of Fries" by Commander Cody. Half a point each for "Hot Dog" by Elvis Presley and "Junk Food Junkie" by Larry Groce. No score for "Slip Slidin' Away" by Paul Simon.

4. (c) 20 percent, according to the National Restaurant Association.

5. The first person to portray Ronald McDonald: Willard Scott.

Don't say cheese. Mmmmm, three ounces of warm, runny cheese between two slices of bread grilled to a golden, greasy brown. Are you really surprised? A grilled cheese sandwich has all the saturated fat of 3½ hot dogs. Without the pleasure of a baseball game.

Convenience Stores

Fresh Ideas for Quick Stops

There are 93,200 convenience stores in the United States. Unless you're on the space shuttle, you probably have easy access to one around the clock.

Yup, that's convenience. But is it the kind of convenience you want? After all, the typical convenience-store customer is a blue-collar guy, ages 18 to 30, dropping by to pick up beer, smokes and a soft drink, according to the National Association of Convenience Stores (NACS). If you'd rather have easy access to vitamins, minerals and fiber, take heart. Convenience-store operators know that more and more people want to feed their bodies well, and proprietors want to make that just as easy as buying a cola and a Moon Pie.

"Men who have been working out or are going to play ball or go running want to watch what they're eating," says Karen Raskopf, a spokeswoman for 7-Eleven, the country's largest convenience-store chain with more than 6,000 outlets.

As long as there's a strong public demand, convenience stores will remain bastions of nutritionally vacant foods, like hot dogs, doughnuts, candy bars, soft drinks and potato chips. But there are alternatives to please the health-conscious buyer in every corner of the store, says Raskopf: pretzels with or without salt, bottled waters, juices, teas, yogurt, frozen yogurt and low-fat granola products, for instance.

Freshness is big, too, opening the door to some low-

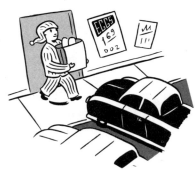

fat, high-carbohydrate eating from your local quick-stop. Twenty-eight percent of all convenience stores in the United States stock some sort of fresh produce, according to the NACS, meaning you can put those Ho Ho's down and pick up a banana as you dash through the aisles.

"I was shocked," says nutritionist Evelyn Tribole. "I was in a 7-Eleven the other day. My heart went pitter-patter. They had fresh fruit—apples and bananas. They had low-fat muffins."

Raskopf said a distribution system that's being phased in at 7-Eleven stores allows daily delivery of such things as fresh produce, sandwiches and baked goods, including bagels and low-fat cream cheese. The company is experimenting in some stores with items like packaged salads, grilled chicken sandwiches and Asian-inspired rice dishes.

Resist Those Impulse Buys

Laudable improvements aside, convenience stores are still no place to give your impulses free rein. Because convenience stores are jam-packed with enticing grab-and-eat foods, you're better off entering with a focused mind, says Dr. Liz Applegate of *Runner's World* magazine.

"You have to decide what it is you're going in there for," Dr. Applegate says. "A lot of people go in to pay for their gas and walk out with one of those disgusting hot dogs because they thought, 'Oh, hey, I'm a little bit hungry.'"

Just as with a burger joint, you should enter with a plan, she says. Need a snack? Make a beeline for the pretzels or low-fat fig bars. Sandwich or burger? Count on the cheaper ones—they're usually lower in fat because they contain less meat. Thirsty? Pick up some orange or grapefruit juice for an extra hit of vitamin C.

Lunch on the Fly

We had heard the rumors: You can actually jog through a convenience store and toss together a somewhat nutritious lunch—something better than a hot dog and a Twinkie, anyway. So we decided to try an experiment at our neighborhood quick-stops: five days, five lunches, for five or six bucks each. All five stores offered sandwiches. The places that sold fresh fruit and low-fat yogurt made life even easier. All the stores offered low-calorie waters, too, but we threw in the occasional juice drink to keep ourselves interested. Ready? Let's do lunch.

7-Eleven

Turkey sub, low-fat blueberry yogurt, Crystal Light raspberry ice drink and a banana

Calories: 795
Fat: 18.5 grams
Cost: $5.26
Comment: Lots of fruit and freshly made sandwiches in a cooler display case.

Uni-Mart

Ham and Swiss sub, Utz "very thin" pretzels (2⅛-ounce bag), black cherry low-fat yogurt, Glacier Ridge raspberry lemonade and an apple

Calories: 1,162
Fat: 17.5 grams
Cost: $5.41
Comment: Our sub was prepared at a deli counter, so we asked for half the regular amount of cheese and only vinegar as a dressing.

Wawa

Ham and cheese sandwich, Katie's Garden Fresh Fruit (plastic container holding 12 ounces of cantaloupe, honeydew melon, pineapple and red grapes) and Boku Seven Fruit Blend drink

Calories: 710
Fat: 16 grams
Cost: $5.77
Comment: Nice selection of fresh fruit. Limited range of pre-made sandwiches, although they also have a deli counter.

Food Mart

Roast beef sandwich, 16 ounces of orange juice, Herr's Bite Size Sourdough Hard Pretzels and a banana

Calories: 926
Fat: 15 grams
Cost: $4.68
Comment: This store is one of those gas station-and-convenience store combinations. We bought here because they had a broader selection of food than many similar operations.

Turkey Hill Minit Market

Turkey sub, Snapple Mango Madness Cocktail and SnackWell's Chocolate Sandwich Cookies

Calories: 760
Fat: 17.5 grams
Cost: $5.37
Comment: Smaller packages of snacks were higher in fat, so we bought a full-size box of Snackwells, ate a couple and stashed the rest in a drawer. No fresh fruit or yogurt available.

Notes: Prices are pre-tax. Nutrition labels on the drinks indicated they held more than one serving. We drank it all in one sitting (wouldn't you?), increasing the calorie count. For food that was missing nutrition labels, we estimated fat and calories from U.S. Department of Agriculture tables and other sources.

In the Car

Cruisin' Cuisine Takes a Turn for the Better

Tail fins, Brylcreem and cheeseburgers. Schoolgirl carhops in little majorette suits who laugh at your jokes 'cause the boss says they have to. One more time around the Char Grill parking lot, then cruise the neon main drag with a tall Dixie cup of soda teetering between the bucket seats. Dang, they keep putting pickles on your burger.

Americans have been drive-through crazy since the 1920s, when Kirby's Pig Stand started vending barbecue sandwiches on the highway between Dallas and Fort Worth—the first restaurant designed for behind-the-wheel dining. There have also been drive-in churches, wedding chapels, funeral parlors and, of course, movies.

But no human function has been so heavily harnessed to the horseless carriage as eating. And lost amid the hubbub of the motorized feeding frenzy was the idea of eating *well*. Since the 1920s, for example, Americans have increased their fat intake by 31 percent.

Now, you're an average guy, right? So you probably drive a little more than 18,000 miles a year. You also take about 50,000 automobile trips in your lifetime, which means you spend an enormous slice of your waking existence out of reach of the nonfat cream cheese you tucked lovingly into the refrigerator.

The good news is that the restaurants lining America's highways are not nearly the nutritional toxic dump that they were just a few years ago. That's the assessment of a guy who

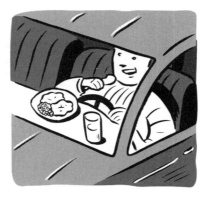

should know—over-the-road truck driver Dave Dobransky of New Albany, Indiana.

"A year ago if you were trying to eat low-fat, it was like a desert out there on the road—you might come to an oasis every once in a long while," says Dobransky, who is renowned in trucking circles for his enthusiasm for healthful eating. "Now some truck stops even offer low-fat options on the menu. For years and years they've been traditionally the trucker type of meal—baked potatoes, meat with gravy and fried foods. But now, the whole industry is starting to modernize."

How to Eat and Run

Okay, Bubba, ready for a road trip? Map, shades, an extra pair of jeans and a dozen CDs. Not bad but, um, how are you with a knife and cutting board?

"Well, what guy is going to get a cooler out and have little plastic bags with fruits and vegetables all cut up and ready to go?" asks Dr. Liz Applegate of *Runner's World* magazine. "Of course that's what somebody might suggest, but the reality is nobody's going to do that. Oh, if that's possible, definitely do it. But if you have a driving partner, if you're giving somebody a ride, say, 'Why don't you bring some fruits and vegetables?' It's worth the suggestion."

Otherwise, Dr. Applegate says, count on pulling off the road for a small meal every three to four hours. "It's good to keep yourself mentally alert," she says. "As blood sugar levels drop, you can lose concentration and get sleepy." Be careful not to stuff yourself, because overeating can make you sleepy, too, she says. And while you're stopping, tank up on fluids so you don't dehydrate. Drink water if you can get it, or diet soda. Just don't overdo it with caffeinated soda.

Speaking of pit stops, you might want to flip back a couple of pages to review the chapter on fast-food restaurants. Then come back here for even more tips about cruisin' cuisine. Go ahead, we'll wait.

Bone up. "You have to be aware of what you're eating on the road," says Dobransky. "Unless you know that a bacon, lettuce and tomato sandwich contains an amount of fat that would just totally blow you away, you're not going to steer away from it." Buy one of those books that lists the fat content of the food offered by chain restaurants, he suggests, and stash it in your glove compartment.

Don't drive bottomless. Suppose you snap open a megabag of cheese curls and prop it in the passenger seat for a highway snack. What's going to happen? The bag will empty out faster than your gas tank. Nutritionist Evelyn Tribole calls that "bottomless eating."

"I look for 'whole' foods, ones that have an end to them, like a bagel, a single-serving packet of pretzels or even little sandwiches. Some of the energy bars are good. I recommend keeping them in your glove box. They seem to last forever. They are pretty forgiving as far as being mushed and crunched." Look for bars that are high in complex carbohydrates, low in fat and made from natural ingredients.

Give nonfat another try. A few nonfat cookies make a mess-free snack for drivers. If you haven't tried them lately, Dobransky says, you might be in for a surprise.

"They came out a few years ago with some nonfat cookies that were the worst thing I've ever eaten in my life," he says. "Hideously bad. But I picked up a package of Archway Fat-Free Sugar Cookies the other day—respectably good. They're not as good as the things Mom

Clean Up Your Juggling Act

How would you feel if someone started juggling hand grenades next to your desk?

Then you can imagine how over-the-road truck driver Dave Dobransky from New Albany, Indiana, feels when he sees you flying down the highway juggling chicken fingers, fries and a shake against the steering wheel. After all, the American Automobile Association says 40 percent of all accidents involve distracted drivers—people who were eating or tuning a radio, for instance.

If you *must* eat while you drive, Dobransky says, choose something that's easy to handle and easy to cast aside in an emergency—a banana, for instance.

The drivers who scare Dobransky most aren't eating at all. "Oh man, you would not believe the near misses that we've had over the years with people on cellular phones," he says. "Their driving abilities just go out the window. It's much more dangerous than eating a banana. I guess it's hard for a person to get that involved with a piece of fruit."

used to bake, but this is a different world now." More of his favorite cab cuisine: bananas, pears, apples, nonfat caramel corn, Louise's Fat-Free potato chips and pretzels.

Cool it. If you're cruising with a cooler, wise use of that in-the-car icebox will liberate you from the nutritional tyranny of fast-food restaurants. Duck into a supermarket for some whole-wheat bread and low-fat lunchmeat. Slap a sandwich together, and put the rest on ice. "While you can go into a burger joint and easily eat something with 26 grams of fat," says Dobransky, "my wife and I literally restrict our intake to 3 grams of fat at lunch."

At the Ballpark

Go Ahead: Get Yer Red Hots

Nearly 100 million people attend professional baseball, basketball and football games in the United States each year. Considering that kind of all-American fervor, it's little wonder that we manage to suck down 581 hot dogs *per second*—more than 18 billion a year.

Now, a run-of-the-mill frankfurter can get 80 percent of its calories from fat, so it's not going to hit any nutritionist's list of top-ten favorites. But if you've forked out good bucks for tickets, shouldered your way through the throng to your seat and, darn it, the experience just isn't the same without a dog and a beer, well, don't get your guilt mechanism revved up. Raise your hand and shout for the vendor. It's not like you do this three times a week.

"What's a ball game without getting a hot dog?" says Dr. Liz Applegate of *Runner's World* magazine. "It's not going to blow your dietary record in the long run, so go ahead and have a good time. But keep it in moderation. You don't want to walk away from the ball game feeling sick because you've had five hot dogs and three buckets of beer."

Hungry? Run for It

If you *wanted* to find something more healthy to eat at a ballpark, could you? You bet, slugger. The first thing you have to do is make a run for it—that is, stand up, head for an exit and find a concession stand. The hawkers who dispense food up and down the aisles of the stadium are not known for their low-fat cuisine.

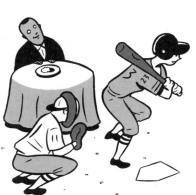

In some ballparks, staffers with handheld computers will come to your seat and take your order. Forget it—do your own walking and burn off a few calories.

Navigating your way to the concession stand may seem like a chore unto itself, but your work is not done. For business reasons, stadium concession stands will probably never be mistaken for a Weight Watchers meeting. But out of the 10 to 15 items you'd find at a typical counter these days, two or three will qualify as healthy eating, says Stephen Beehag, who manages food development for Sportservice, which dishes out the food at seven major-league parks.

"The whole business is changing," says Beehag, a former chef. "It certainly isn't the pizza, hot dog and nacho business that it was. I'm not saying those items have declined, but there is a lot of enthusiasm when we put other items out there, like healthy salads with grilled chicken on top and the dressing on the side."

Even among the traditional offerings, you can find some low-fat snacks, points out Dr. Applegate—unbuttered popcorn, for instance, and licorice whips.

What other products are worth taking a swing at? Here's a sampling of some healthful offerings that are popping up in ballparks around the country. Not all ballparks serve these foods, but you may find some of them on the menu at a ballpark near you.

- Rotisserie chicken: A reasonable alternative to fried chicken. But it's still a good idea to remove the skin.
  - Meatless chili: With artful spicing, you'll never miss the beef.
  - Vegetarian burritos: Crammed with zucchini strips, peppers and onions on a flour tortilla.
  - Sliced turkey sandwiches.
  - Veggie plates: Fresh cucumbers, celery, carrots and radishes.
  - Fresh juices and mineral water: An alternative to beer.

A Brief History of Tubesteak

Hot dogs and other sausages have been in and out of hot water since ancient times.

It was 3,500 years B.T.C. (Before Ty Cobb) when the Babylonians got the novel idea of spicing meat, stuffing it into an animal's intestine and then eating it. An idea like that is bound to spread. By the eighth century B.C. Homer was lusting over fire-roasted sausages. Things simmered along tastily in the ancient world until those rowdy Romans and their fermented grapes got involved.

Toga! Toga!

It's not clear precisely how wieners fit into the equation, but the pagan feast of Lupercalia was a notoriously drunken and gluttonous festival that included sexual initiation rites. Constantine the Great, the first Christian emperor, was so shocked by these toga parties that he banned the holiday *and* sausages. Draw your own conclusions.

When European colonists arrived in North America, they found that sausage had already staked a claim. Native Americans were making their own version out of chopped meat and dried berries, which was smoked and stored for later consumption.

But sausage really came into its own in the United States during the Industrial Revolution, when European immigrants flocked into the country with their Old World recipes. Around the beginning of the twentieth century, sausage became America's original fast food. Vendors would sell their greasy delicacies to passersby and, to prevent the drippings from ruining customers' clothes, they wrapped each in a bun.

How the Dog Got Its Name

Legend has it that the opening day of baseball season was particularly cold in 1900 at the Polo Grounds in New York City, so the food-service folk were sent into the stands barking a pitch for "red-hot" dachshund sausages, as they were called. An amused newspaper cartoonist, T. A. Dorgan, recorded the practice by depicting actual yappy little dogs stuffed into buns. In lieu of the cumbersome word dachshund, he labeled the bowsers "hot dogs." Thus the modern-day term.

But gloom once again descended on the world of wieners as the term hot dog brought disrepute to the popular snack. Persistent rumors about bowwow meat making its way into the sausage casing caused no end of distress in Coney Island, a hotbed of hot dog sales. In 1913 the chamber of commerce there banned use of the term on signs and menus. There is no record of their opinion of toga parties.

Still, they might have been on to something. If the ban had stuck, we all could have been spared the 1984 release of *Hot Dog: The Movie.*

On an Airplane

You're in the Control Tower

You reserved your seat on the airplane. You reserved a ride on the limo. You reserved a rental car at your destination and a hotel bed with Magic Fingers. But did you reserve your food?

Yes, it's time to stop complaining about airline food. With little extra effort you can arrange for the flight attendant to deliver a meal that fits your nutritional specifications. The less savvy passengers will wonder how you merit special treatment. No need to tell 'em it comes at no extra cost. No need to tell 'em you just spoke up when you booked your seat.

"Most airlines that serve meals will also have special meals that are low-fat, vegetarian and—one of my favorites—seafood," says nutritionist Evelyn Tribole.

Swissair, for instance, offers more than 30 variations you can pick from at the time you make your reservation or up to 24 hours in advance. They offer low-calorie, low-fat, low-protein, nonlactose, high-fiber, low-fiber and bland dinners (we know what you're thinking, but these are *really* bland dinners, for people who have trouble stomaching spices). There also are meals for vegetarians, babies, children, people with diabetes and people who follow religious restrictions.

"I don't think airline food will ever be anything that we'll look forward to, but do make the healthier choices," adds Agnes Kolor, R.D., a Pearl River, New York, nutritionist who consulted for Oprah Winfrey's television show. "Try to choose meals that aren't fried or have a lot of batter and added fat."

Before You Call the Cab . . .

As long as you're making plans for sound eating during a flight, here are other easy steps to take before you head for the airport.

Get hotel help. You've seen the best food the airlines have to offer and it isn't good enough. Who ya gonna call? Room service! That's right, lots of hotels these days offer exotic boxed lunches that are made just for tossing into a flight bag. So next time you have to fly, call the hotel desk and tell them you want one for the road.

Go bananas. Take matters into your own hands. In your carry-on luggage pack a healthy snack, like fruit, a bagel or a one-serving box of cereal. Then you'll be able to wave off the smoked almonds when the drink cart gets rolling.

Travel light. Say you're flying to the home office. You want to be able to tap-dance freshly into the terminal where your boss is waiting to take you to dinner. "Order a fruit plate for the flight," suggests Dr. Liz Applegate of *Runner's World* magazine. "This way you're probably going to get less than 200 calories, depending on the airline. You've had something to eat and you feel refreshed. You've had fiber, potassium, the whole bit. You get off the plane feeling crisp. You can go to dinner and not feel like you've sat on the plane and eaten that questionable chicken dish."

Try automatic pilot. If a secretary or travel agent makes all of your flight reservations, ask that person to keep a record of your food requirements, Dr. Applegate suggests. Every time they make a reservation for you, they can automatically order your special dinner, too. All you have to do is mention it the first time.

Pass on the gas. Ever buy a bag of pretzels at a low elevation and then drive into the mountains? The air inside the

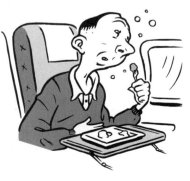

sealed bag expands at the higher altitude, making it puff up like a cellophane blowfish. How do you feel about replaying that experiment with your gastrointestinal tract? You might, if you eat gas-causing foods, like cantaloupe, watermelon, honeydew melon or carbonated drinks, just before or during a flight, says Maria Simonson, Sc.D., Ph.D, director of the Health, Weight and Stress Clinic at Johns Hopkins Medical Institutions in Baltimore.

She notes that it would be wise to avoid greasy food, too much food of any kind and carbonated drinks on the day of your flight. Dr. Simonson suggests that you stick to fruit juices or noncarbonated beverages.

It's Never Too Late

Maybe planning is not your forte. You forgot to bring a book to read, you forgot to pack extra underwear and you forgot to order a low-fat meal for your plane trip. That doesn't mean your fate is sealed once you hit the terminal. Here are ways to get a nutritional edge during your flight.

Search the cupboards. If the dinner being passed around the cabin sets off your fat alarm, talk to the flight attendant. Chances are there's something else available on the airplane—commonly a cold platter of some kind or fruit. There's even a chance your airline carries the same kind of frozen low-fat dinners you buy in the supermarket.

Stay fluid. All that dry air rushing around the cabin of an airplane is sucking water right out of your body, which can leave you cranky and fatigued, says Dr. Applegate. In a three-hour flight, you can easily lose more than a pint of water just through your skin and by

breathing. We know what you're thinking, but alcohol only dehydrates you more. Same with coffee. Ask for lots of bottled water.

How Food Takes Flight

Just how does that little plate of Chicken Surprise end up on your fold-down table at 30,000 feet? To find out, we collared Ingrid Moughal, who develops food concepts for Swissair. Here's how airlines work their food magic.

First, go shopping. Oh, the food you'd need to feed 2,000 clients a day in North America wouldn't quite fit into a grocery cart. But Moughal does cruise supermarkets and specialty stores for inspiration. She especially likes health food stores and reads health and nutrition newsletters for tips. She also scouts out recipes that will adapt to airline food service.

Get a plan. Foods that work well together are worked into a menu—first course, entrée, salad and dessert. After checking with the home office, Moughal sends this information around to the airline's caterers.

See if it flies. The caterers prepare the food as described and hold presentations where airline sales staffers, crew members, customers and journalists critique the presentation and taste. Adjustments are made if necessary.

Get cooking. Within a few months the caterers start preparing meals to the new specifications. Most caterers, situated close to airports, service more than one airline. The food is loaded onto the airline's equipment, trucked to the airport and put onto your airplane.

Pass out the silverware. Because the caterers prepare meals in stages, it's hard to pinpoint how long before departure your meal was cooked. Call it two to ten hours.

At the Bar

Eat, Drink and Be Merry

It's tough to hoist an after-work brew without getting nutritionally mugged. As any watering-hole wiseman can tell you, the usual pattern can be broken down to the three stages of intoxication.

1. Let's have a drink at the bar before dinner.
2. One more round. Then we'll eat.
3. To hell with dinner.

Taverns are a kind of nutritional vortex. You have a drink and, hey, there's a bowl of nuts on the bar. With your thirst freshly salted, you signal the barkeep for another drink. Around and around you go until, whoa, you ain't in Kansas anymore, Toto.

If this sounds familiar to you, now is the time to come to the aid of your body. Okay, maybe your role model is Norm on *Cheers* and you really do like hanging out at a place where everybody knows your name. Fine. After all, George Wendt—the actor who played Norm on the hit series—was an avid runner at the time. If you apply some body science, some common sense and some moderation, you'll be able to take a seat at the tavern without having to worry about leaving a permanent indentation.

Eat first. If you drink on an empty stomach, the alcohol will affect you more quickly. You want to have fun in a bar, not be lobotomized. Besides, if you go to a bar hungry, you'll start sucking down fatty, salty appetizers that do your body little good—Buffalo wings, meatballs, cocktail weenies, chips, cheese and potato skins.

"If you're meeting the guys after work and it's going to roll through dinnertime, try to

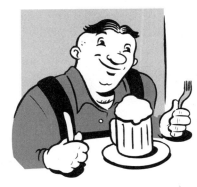

get something to eat at four o'clock," says Dr. Liz Applegate of *Runner's World* magazine. "You know, stop at the vending machine at the office and get an apple, a carton of yogurt—something low-fat. But don't go to a bar starving."

Make your bar a watering hole. You can temper the negative effects of drinking alcohol—not only intoxication but dehydration, too—by working in some water now and then. Between beers, ask the saloon keeper for a mineral water with a twist or a club soda. If you alternate alcoholic drinks with water, you cut your caloric and alcohol consumption in half, says nutritionist Evelyn Tribole.

Lick the salt habit. If you're going to eat in a bar, find something that's low-salt, like cut-up vegetables. If you crunch down those salty pretzels, corn chips and nachos, you'll end up drinking more than you intended.

"The bar is kind of playing you, you know?" says nutritionist Agnes Kolor. "You're walking into their trap, eating all of their salty foods so you'll need more of their drinks."

How Drinking Goes to Waist

This is an age when the money college students spend on alcohol far exceeds the cost of running college libraries.

Boy, do we guzzle the calories. And when you drink alcohol, you get girth along with the mirth. Dietary surveys estimate that drinkers get 5 to 20 percent of their total energy from alcohol, or 100 to 600 calories a day. And 3 percent of all people over age 15 get more than 1,000 calories a day from alcohol.

Well, you could just reduce the calories you get from other sources, right?

No. An approach like that would rob you of vital nutrition. "Alcohol is very high in calories, and there's no nutritional value," Kolor says. "It doesn't mean you can't have a drink here or there.

When You Belly Up to the Bar

It's not only alcoholic beverages that pad your midsection. Those bowls and bags of over-the-counter snack foods do their part, too. Here's a rundown of what you're getting in some common bar fare.

Bar Food	Calories	Fat (g.)	Sodium (mg.)
Buffalo wings, 7	736	44	1,585
Cashews, 1 oz.	163	13.2	182
Cheese crackers, 1 oz.	134	6	290
Mixed nuts, 1 oz.	169	14.6	190
Nachos, cheese, 6 to 8	346	19	816
Nachos, supreme, 6 to 8	569	30.7	1,800
Peanuts, 1 oz.	164	13.9	123
Pistachios, 1 oz.	164	13.7	222
Potato sticks, 1 oz.	148	9.8	71
Pretzels, 1 oz.	125	1.4	538
Tortilla chips, 1 oz.	150	8	155

But you're getting a lot of empty calories—and by empty I mean non-nutritious calories. No bang for your buck."

Besides, the calories in alcohol don't satisfy your appetite. Researchers at Laval University in Quebec City, Quebec, monitored the food intake of eight men who were allowed to eat freely and drink beer during four two-day sessions in a laboratory. They didn't tell the guys, but half of the time they were drinking alcohol-free beer. (No word on whether they sued.) The men were fed a different diet each session, too: low-fat food and alcohol-free beer, low-fat food with alcohol, high-fat food and no alcohol and high-fat food with alcohol.

The researchers' conclusion: Your hunger mechanism is blind to alcohol. So when you drink, you gain seven calories for each gram of alcohol and you don't compensate by eating less. That means it's more likely you'll gain pounds, particularly if you're also eating a high-fat diet. A larger study, using 351 men and 360 women, confirmed those results.

So if you had doubts before, there's your proof: Drinking is fattening. But how fast can the lard pile up? Suppose you drank two regular beers a day but didn't compensate by eating less or by exercising more. You'd gain a pound every ten days.

Check Your Math

Any drinker worth his margarita salt knows that one or two drinks a day can actually lower your risk of heart disease. Careful, though, that benefit is easy to wipe out: Heavy drinking contributes to high blood pressure, which greatly increases your risk of heart disease.

A study that tracked 1,455 men for 12 years found that their blood pressure rose steadily if they drank more than six beers a week.

So let's be sure we're counting drinks correctly: One drink means a standard 12-ounce can of beer, a 4- to 6-ounce glass of wine or one jigger of hard alcohol.

At the Party

Celebrate without Gaining Weight

Which sounds like more fun to you?

- Lolling in a hammock or wearing a strait-jacket?
- Hiking through the woods or walking on a treadmill in a dingy basement?
- Grazing your way through a holiday buffet or biting your tongue and pretending that a tantalizing table full of food is a cruel illusion?

Last time we consulted with Merriam Webster, the words *celebration* and *holiday* had a lot to do with fun and merriment. And not much to do with the Marquis de Sade. By their very nature, special occasions only come up once in a long while—which means that eating party food moderately is not going to prompt your waistband and shirt buttons to dial 911.

Now, ponder the word *moderate*. Tell yourself that you're going to have a gleeful romp through the taste treats but that you're not going to totally pig out in the process. After all, the third sugar-covered rum ball tastes pretty much like the second one you ate, so there's no need to keep popping them into your maw. Move along, little doggie—find something new to sample.

"Not only does alcohol have a lot of calories, but research shows that it may impact fat metabolism—making it harder for fat to get burned," says nutritionist Evelyn Tribole. "Drinking can also cause you to forget to think about what you're eating. You know: 'Ahh, who cares?' I try to alternate drinks with nonalcoholic,

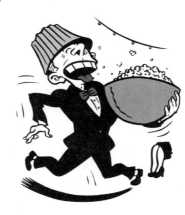

noncaloric beverages, like sparkling water."

Alcohol also interferes with your vitamin and mineral metabolism, causes fluid loss and, of course, dilutes your IQ. So if you're going to drink, doctors say, keep it to no more than one or two a day.

Before the Bash

Took a shower? Check.

Skimmed the newspaper so you'll make intelligent conversation? Check.

Slipped on some casually elegant duds that have seen the inside of a washing machine in recent weeks? Check.

Then it's party time, right?

Well, keep your toga on, Claudius. We have a couple of pre-party maneuvers that will temper your feeding instincts.

Launch a pre-emptive snack. There's an old rule stating that you should never go to the grocery store hungry. "The same thing applies to parties," says nutritionist Agnes Kolor. "Never go to a party on an empty stomach." Before attending a recent wedding, Kolor had a piece of fruit. "I still ate at the wedding and I had a great time," she says. But she wasn't famished and she avoided overeating.

If you're planning to head straight from work to some bacchanalia, toss salt-free pretzels or a banana into your briefcase for an afternoon snack, Kolor suggests. You'll arrive at the party with a tamed appetite. Then you can try out some opening lines on the guests rather than elbowing your way to the bowl of chocolate truffles.

Bring your own. Stack the deck in your favor. Take along a party food that you know fits into your eating plan, like salsa and nonfat tortilla chips or a vegetable plate with yogurt dip.

Beware Automatic Eating

The party's popping. You're in midsentence, making a penetrating point about international politics to this striking stranger who actually thinks you know what you're talking about. But you stop, puzzled to be tasting nachos in your mouth. You look down and see a hand—your hand—directing another greasy cheese-and-beef monster toward your lips.

Brain to hand, brain to hand: That nacho is not cleared to land. Repeat: NOT cleared to land.

"I tell people not to stand right beside the snack table or the appetizer table," says Kolor. "You'll be talking. Your hand just reaches down—it's an unconscious motion. You're constantly eating. You have more control if you go get a plate and put the food on it and move away from the buffet."

Here are other ways to impose a little decorum before the whole buffet spread goes marching into your gullet.

Talk it out. When you enter the room, strike up a conversation with someone right away. Remember, this is a social occasion. There's plenty of time to work your way to the trough.

Do reconnaissance. Before you start snatching up cocktail weenies from the appetizer table, scope out the whole spread. First time through, stock your little party plate with low-fat munchies, like pretzels, fruit and sliced vegetables.

Go limp. Trade in that Chinet plate for a flimsy little cocktail napkin. You'll be less inclined to pile it up into a handheld smorgasbord. If each foray to the buffet table nets you a single little morsel on your napkin, your eating will be much more measured.

Set priorities. Gravitate toward the foods that have some special significance— unique holiday cookies, for example, or the spinach torte that Charlie's been bragging about all year. Forget the mixed nuts—you can get them anywhere. And remember that eating at a buffet table is not a timed event, so you can take it easy. Savor the stuff you really like, then back away.

Belts That Are a Notch Above

At times of merriment, by golly, you want a drink. And no stranger speaking from the pages of a book is going to persuade you otherwise. Fine. Here are some smart choices among popular holiday drinks.

- **Beer:** A better choice than the hard stuff since it's higher in carbohydrates. Just the process of digesting a beer burns off nearly a quarter of its calories. If you're going to have more than one, find one with the word "light" on the label. They run about 100 calories.
- **Bloody Mary:** About 115 calories and less than a gram of fat.
- **Champagne:** Cheers—just 84 calories per flute.
- **Rum toddy:** A reasonable choice at 114 calories a glass. The hot water, nutmeg, sugar and lemon slice will make you feel fuller and less inclined to stuff yourself.
- **White wine spritzer:** 70 calories.

And a few to avoid:

- **Eggnog:** Why suck down an extra ten grams of fat and 171 calories when you don't really like the stuff anyway? The same goes for other cream-based drinks, like White Russians.
- **Daiquiri:** 224 calories.
- **Dessert wines:** 157 calories per glass. If you love this stuff, go ahead. But if somebody's just passing it around to spread holiday cheer, ask yourself: Isn't there something I'd rather be drinking?

Toss your empties. Once you've cleared your appetizer plate, drop it into the trash bin right away. If you stand around holding it, more food will undoubtedly materialize on it.

A Holiday Sampler

Not every party treat is going to launch you into cardiac arrest from fat overload. Around Thanksgiving, for instance, you'll find tons of cancer-fighting beta-carotene in pumpkin pie and breads made with winter squashes.

"And definitely go for the shrimp. Those are the lowest in fat and the best tasting—that's my bias," says Tribole.

"Usually there are cut-up vegetables, breadsticks or rolls," adds Kolor. "Now, mozzarella sticks or Buffalo wings are going to be high in fat—but it's fine to have that, too. You just want to have a balance between the lower-fat, lower-sodium foods and the higher-fat, higher-sodium foods."

Here's a nutritional rundown of many culinary stalwarts you'll find at a party buffet.

Do the funky chicken. Not the dance, unless it's a 1960s theme party. Sliced chicken breast, though, is always a good move, at 141 calories and three grams of fat for a three-ounce portion. Another sure bet: One large steamed shrimp has 5 calories and nearly zip for fat.

Sliced pork, on the other hand, weighs in at 177 calories and eight grams of fat per portion. And forget the unidentifiable processed meats—each ounce carries 80 to 100 calories and eight or nine grams of fat.

There oughtta be a slaw. With a sizable dose of mayo, potato salad will deliver 179 calories and ten grams of fat per half-cup. Reach for the coleslaw instead—41 calories and two grams of fat per half-cup.

Beware of spreadable edibles. Got a choice of pâtés? You won't find a low-fat liver spread, but if it's from a chicken, you're talking about 58 percent of calories from fat; for goose it's 85 percent of the calories from fat. The difference is something to cluck about.

What about the requisite cheese log? Seventy-five percent of its calories are from fat.

Dip: If it's cream-cheese-based, it has 100 calories and ten grams of fat per ounce (about a tablespoon). Hint: To trim fat, dip with vegetables instead of chips.

Guacamole: Two grams of fat in a tablespoon.

Fudge a little. Don't make a meal of the chocolate-covered almonds and peanuts—160 calories per ounce, with 12 grams of fat. A single brownie with nuts: 300 calories and 21 grams of fat. By comparison, that makes fudge a splendid choice: 112 calories and 3 grams of fat per ounce.

Skinny Dipping

There's nothing like getting a bunch of your best buds together to watch the big game. And that's fine, provided you exercise first and nosh on some low-fat snacks during the event. There are plenty of low-fat dips on the market now, but if you're scooping them up with greasy potato chips, you're not exactly doing your heart any favors. So the next time you host a bash, or just have to bring something, keep in mind these heart-healthy suggestions from world-famous chef Jacques Pépin for stuff you can dip.

- **A pleasing pepper platter.** Slice and arrange raw orange, red, yellow, purple and green peppers.
- **Jícama.** Peel and cut into sticks or rounds. This root vegetable has a sweet, crunchy taste, like an apple.
- **Celery root** (also called celeriac). Pungent celery relative; peel and cut into sticks. (To prevent browning, dip in water with a little lemon juice.)
- **Endive leaves.** Each makes a little scoop, with a slightly bitter flavor.

At the Movies

No Need to Be Afraid

Gulp. That cute teenager up on the screen is settling back onto the bed, eyelids drooping. Any second now dream-monster Freddy Krueger is going to slash out of the mattress and chop her into sushi. Your own hand is in overdrive delivering popcorn to your mouth. Chomp, chomp, chomp. Gulp.

There's something insidious lurking in the dark, all right. Yow! It's right in your lap! Your bucket of popcorn! Why, it's pumping sickening gunk into your bloodstream that's going to choke your heart!

Relax. We're going to show you how to fight back.

Most moviegoers buy snacks, and most of those snack buyers go for popcorn. The problem is that movie popcorn is prepared in a number of ways, and some of those methods wallop you with saturated fat or trans fatty acids, the kind that clog your arteries. When the *Nutrition Action Healthletter* folks analyzed popcorn from six chains across the country, they found that the average large plain order had two days' worth of heart-damaging fat. Ask for some butterlike-flavoring substance and you might as well eat nine Quarter Pounders.

There's a happy plot twist: Their report fired a revolution in theaters. Many dumped the harmful coconut oil or partially hydrogenated vegetable oil they had used. The changeover wasn't unanimous, however, so you still need to check at the counter. Here are the common popping methods.

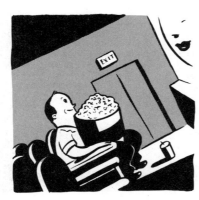

- Air popping. Two thumbs up for this low-fat method. Get it without butter and eat as much as you want. After all, you're getting loads of fiber.
- Nonhydrogenated vegetable oil. You'll still get lots of fat, but not the nastiest stuff, saturated and trans fats.
- Partially hydrogenated vegetable shortening. High in trans fats, which will line your arteries.
- Coconut oil. Two thumbs down. Heart attack in a bucket.

If you don't like your theater's popping technique, speak up. Tell the clerk. Tell the manager. Call their corporate offices.

"I think the movie theater popcorn study was probably the best example of how much power consumers have to change an industry," says Jayne Hurley of the Center for Science in the Public Interest. "Within weeks of our study coming out the theaters started popping in healthier oils."

Heroic Proportions

What is it about the movies that makes everything larger than life? We don't mean John Wayne. We're talking about candy bars the size of a multiplex screen. Whatever you haul into the theater is likely to be eaten before Freddy slices up his third teenager. So use some portion control at the outset.

"Some theaters offer candy by the bulk, so you can buy smaller amounts as opposed to monster size," says nutritionist Evelyn Tribole. "Then you aren't obligating yourself to a five-pound candy bar."

If you must have candy, remember that some are kinder to the heart than others. Look for candy that's non- or lower-fat rather than a sugar-and-fat combo. Licorice, hard candy and chocolate-covered nougats, caramels and mints are better, therefore, than solid chocolate or chocolate-covered peanut butter with nuts.

On the Trail

Tell Fat to Take a Hike

Grunting and groaning through the wilderness like a pack mule is not recreation. When you're hiking, you want the experience to be like, well, a stroll in the country.

You might know instinctively to leave your boccie ball set at home, but feeding yourself properly while hiking is a trickier matter, even if you're just on the trail for a day or two. As always, you want energy from your food, but you also want it to be lightweight, compact, durable, tasty and easy to prepare.

"The whole idea when you're hiking is to eat low-fat, high-carbohydrate food, to give you sustained energy," says Dr. Liz Applegate of *Runner's World* magazine. This means plenty of fruits, vegetables and grain foods.

Trail food rule number one is to pick lightweight, calorie-dense foods, preferably ones that have had some of their water removed. Modern hikers also have a wide array of featherweight equipment available, including resealable plastic freezer bags (they're tougher than regular resealable bags), squeeze tubes for peanut butter or mustard (fill them from the end and clip them closed), spice shakers and plastic containers for liquids.

A Backpacker's Buffet

Here are some food ideas that are guaranteed to have you singing around the campfire.

Don't be so fresh. For once, fresh might not be the best. Imagine a banana after two days of bouncing. Besides, fresh foods weigh more because they're often high in water content. Eat your fresh foods first to

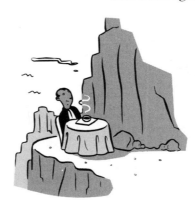

lighten your load and prevent spoilage.

Can it. For perishable protein-rich foods, like tuna, chicken or other meats, consider cans. The good news is that they're inexpensive, they come in a zillion varieties and they last longer than you'd ever want to be on the trail. The bad news is that they're heavy, since they contain lots of water, and you have to carry those cans back to civilization.

Get dehydrated. Dehydrated foods, such as raisins and dried apples and peaches, have much of the water sucked out of them, so they're lighter and won't spoil.

Dry out. Dried foods are lightweight and make up a major part of the veteran backpacker's diet—powdered milk, eggs and cheese, dried vegetables (mushrooms, onions and potatoes), grains (rice and oatmeal), beans, lentils, teas, juices, powdered soups and sauces—and most are available in your local supermarket.

Buy freeze-dried. Soak these lightweight packages in water, or cook them a little while, and foop, they're just like the fresh original. Choose from berries, pears, corn, carrots, chicken, tuna, eggs, cottage cheese and even entrées, like shrimp Creole. They're more expensive than the products you can buy at the supermarket and are found only at backpacking or camping supply stores or from mail-order houses.

Mix it up. Many of the commercial "trail mix" snacks you'll find contain high-fat items that work against you, says nutritionist Evelyn Tribole. "Granola has changed a lot," she says, "and now you can get a low-fat granola easily. But the problem with trail mix is that there are a lot of nuts and seeds and coconut. You are getting a lot of fat."

The solution? Buy some trail mix but doctor it up with high-energy ingredients, like raisins, dried apricots and pretzels. Or mix up your own from scratch, going light on the nuts.

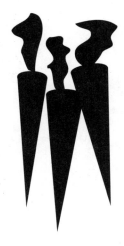

Part Four

Eating for Purpose

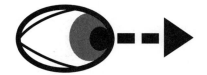

Great Sex

Savoring the Fruits of Passion

When you first met her, you got turned on by watching the way she wiped the spaghetti sauce off the corner of her lip. Just hearing her ask you to pass the peas sent chills down your spine. You were like Jack Nicholson and Jessica Lange in the steamy, kitchen love scene from *The Postman Always Rings Twice*, smashing dishes in a wild frenzy of passion. It was that great.

Now, the thrill is gone. Each day you eat, not necessarily together. Then you lay on the couch and watch the evening prime time lineup. She reads women's magazines with articles like "87 Things That Are Better Than Sex." Every once in a while you glance at one another and both silently think, "Maybe tomorrow."

It's time to bring food back into your sex life.

"If you are well-fed, you are more likely to think about sex than if you are not well-fed," says George Armelagos, Ph.D., professor of anthropology at Emory University in Atlanta and author of *Consuming Passions*.

Eating for Pleasure

When most guys think about food and sex, the first thing that probably springs to mind is whipped cream. That's not what we're talking about here.

But stay with us. We will get to that later. We're talking about ways you can eat smarter for more sensational sex, because when you get right down to it, the food you put *in* your body is ultimately more important for sex than the food you smear *on* her body. Here

are some helpful hints.

Make a B-line. The B vitamins thiamin, riboflavin and niacin are all needed for a healthy sex drive. If you drink alcohol on a daily basis, you may want to take a daily 100 milligram thiamin supplement, because alcohol depletes that vitamin. Otherwise, you can get it by eating whole grains, asparagus and raw nuts. Riboflavin is found in asparagus, bananas, broccoli and lean meats.

Niacin dilates blood vessels, creating better blood flow, and it also synthesizes sex hormones. But if you take it in supplement form, it can irritate your stomach, causing ulcers. It's found in fish, lean meats, peas and beans.

C about a supplement. Vitamin C helps keep your various sex glands running smoothly and your skin smooth and elastic. It also keeps sperm strong by protecting them against free radicals that make them cling together in immobile clumps. Vitamin C is found in citrus fruits, strawberries, kiwifruit, tomatoes and green vegetables. Taking a 250 milligram supplement a day may improve your sperm's chances of fertilizing an egg.

Dial E for excitement. Vitamin E aids sex hormone production and improves circulation. Be careful about taking large doses, however, because it can increase blood pressure. If you are taking supplements, start below 100 international units. It is naturally found in nuts, seeds, beans, whole grains, fruits and vegetables.

Be Zeus with zinc. The body needs 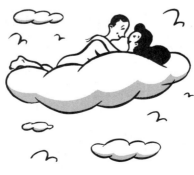 zinc to produce testosterone, the male sex hormone. It also increases sperm production and the volume of ejaculate and may protect sperm from vaginal bacteria. Either too little or too much zinc can negatively affect your sex drive. You can easily get your Daily Value of 15 milligrams by eating steamed oysters, pumpkin seeds, sunflower seeds, garlic and spinach.

Foods of Love

Many items considered as aphrodisiacs work for a very simple reason: because you believe they will. Your brain is your biggest sex organ. If it thinks something turns you into a love machine, it will, says Dr. Armelagos. So if you believe salted crackers will fire up your libido, chances are they will, he says.

Some aphrodisiacs—such as oysters—work because they contain nutrients that your body needs. But they only work if your body needs those nutrients. Oysters are packed with zinc, so if you are zinc deficient, oysters may help you feel sexy. If you're not zinc deficient and oysters make you feel sexy, it's probably your brain doing all the work, Dr. Armelagos says.

There is scientific evidence to back up some other aphrodisiacs. Here are a few.

• Caffeine. Daily coffee drinkers are almost twice as likely to describe themselves as sexually active. And coffee-drinking men report fewer erection problems. "Some caffeine will wake you up. If you feel sluggish and caffeine wakes you up, then you're going to say, 'Oh, I'm horny,' instead of saying, 'Oh, I'm going to go back to sleep,'" says Jeanne Shaw, Ph.D., a certified sex therapist and clinical psychologist in Atlanta.

Once you move beyond moderate drinking, though—a couple of cups a day—you can reverse the effect. Too much caffeine can make you so hyper that you can't focus on feeling turned on.

• Chocolate. It has a number of ingredients that make us feel good. The stimulants theobromine and caffeine get our hearts beating. And a component called phenylethylalanine is thought to produce an "in-love sensation" that dulls pain.

Stump the Sexperts: The Quiz

Think you know a lot about sex? Let's see how you do on this quiz. Then turn the page for the answers.

1. **Which of the following has at some point during history been used to perk up a man's penis?**
(a) Beheading a male partridge and having the doctor eat the heart and the patient drink the bird's blood mixed with water; (b) Smearing oil, pepper and nettleseed on a dildo and sticking it up the anus; (c) Eating hippopotamus snout; (d) Eating hyena eyes; (e) All of the above.

2. **What food did the ancient Egyptians mold into the shape of a penis and why?**

3. **The sea slug has been considered an aphrodisiac by the Arabs and Chinese partly because it displays a trait that is similiar to the male penis. What is it?**

4. **What animal was used to make Spanish fly?**

5. **Which of the following is a man more likely to do after having sex?** (a) Get something to eat; (b) Have a beer; (c) Smoke a cigarette.

Bonus question: When the Aborigines of central Australia ask "Utna ilkukabaka?" it can mean one of two things. One is, "Have you eaten?" What's the other?

• Celery. If you want her to crave you instead of a magazine, this is what you want to eat. Androsterone, a potent male hormone, is thought to attract females, and it can be found in celery. Researchers speculate that when you eat celery, you can release the androsterone through perspiration after digestion. The woman can't actually smell it consciously, but she'll want to get her nose near your skin.

• Pumpkin pie. You don't have to eat it. Just bake it. Researchers at the Smell and Taste Treatment and Research Foundation in Chicago measured blood flow to the penises of 31 men as they smelled different scents. The combination of pumpkin pie and lavender really got the blood moving. Other penis picker-uppers

Stump the Sexperts: The Answers

If you're just browsing, turn back a page to find the "Stump the Sexperts" quiz. No fair peeking at the answers below.

1. **(e).**
2. **Bread. In his book,** *Consuming Passions,* **Emory University's Dr. Armelagos says the Egyptians may have made the association between bread and the male sex organ because bread swells as it bakes.**
3. **It swells and grows when touched.**
4. **Also known as cantharides, Spanish fly was made from a beetle found in southern Europe. The bug was dried and pulverized. When eaten, it irritated the gastrointestinal system and dilated blood vessels, causing erections of the penis or clitoris. The bug's damage to the kidneys, though, was fatal in some cases.**
5. **(a). About 6.8 percent of men usually eat after sex, compared with 5.7 percent who have a drink and 3.4 percent who smoke.**

Bonus question: "Have you had sexual intercourse?"

include doughnut combined with black licorice, pumpkin pie combined with doughnut and plain old orange.

• Serotonin. It's a chemical that your brain produces when you eat a food that contains the amino acid tryptophan along with some carbohydrates. Low levels of serotonin have been linked to low sperm count, poor ejaculation and low virility. Stress will deplete serotonin. But when you eat the tryptophan-carbohydrate combination, it calms you down and replaces the needed serotonin to boost your sexual desire. Try combining about 3.5 ounces of fish, poultry or lean beef with bread or pasta.

A Menu for Love

There's a reason watching her wipe spaghetti sauce off of her lip turned you on a year ago but now barely distracts you from thinking about what's on TV tonight. When you first met, your body produced chemicals that put you happily in love. Then it stopped. You can't turn back the clock, but you can make dinner more sensual.

Reserve a table for two. First of all, to have a sexy dinner, you need to see each other while you eat. Often couples are too busy to eat together. "Dual career couples who don't have time for each other are stressing their own growth by not having some ritual in the day when they are together," says Dr. Shaw. "Dining together is a ritual that has more nutrition in it than just the food."

Have a slow hand. One of the worst sex sappers is stress, and if you wolf down your meal, it contributes to stress. So take it easy. Chew. Taste. Savor it.

Feed each other. Need we say more?

Pass the salt. Throughout the meal, do little things that will warm her heart. "These little acts of kindness at the dinner table really create feelings of warmth and unity and enhance feelings of sexuality later in the evening," says Doreen Virtue, Ph.D., a relationship expert and psychologist in Anaheim, California, and author of *In the Mood.* Don't wait for your mate to ask you to pass the salt or whatever other seasoning she usually uses. Offer it to her without being asked. If you've been paying attention at all, you know what she likes. If you haven't been paying attention, start. Now.

Cooperate, don't criticize. It's good

A Taste of Love

Okay. We promised we'd get to the whipped cream part. And here it is. The problem is that real whipped cream and other foods can possibly cause bacterial infections if they get into your lover's private parts. So what's a horny and hungry guy to do? Try some fun food products specifically made for love. Being the tireless workaholics we are, we called a bunch of sex toy distributors and had them send us edible items for a taste test. Here's what we found.

What's Hot

Choca-Nuki Massage Lotion

It has a slight chocolate taste but only about four calories per gram. Heats up when massaged or blown on. The only drawbacks: It's not chocolate and too much can make the chocolatee feel like a candy apple.

Naked and Naughty Chocolate Finger Paint

Comes in dark and white chocolate flavors. Both taste great though the dark tastes better. One tablespoon packs 3.5 grams of fat, 50 calories and 2.5 grams of cholesterol. Keep it away from female genitals to avoid infection.

My Joy Body Gel

The next best thing to eating Jell-O in bed. No fat or calories. Sticks to body better than Jell-O would, but has slight chemical taste.

What's Not

Doc Johnson Strawberry Body Jam

Not sticky. No calories. Yucky, artificial aftertaste. Smells like Silly Putty.

Doc Johnson Body Pudding

No fat or calories. Smells like it's going to taste good. But be forewarned: It doesn't taste like it smells. It's like eating face cream mixed with Anbesol.

Kingman Industries Edible Undies

No fat or calories. Tastes like a Fruit Roll-Up gone bad. Sticks to roof of mouth and turns skin pink.

Doc Johnson Peaches 'n' Cream Body Butter

No fat or calories. Looks, smells and tastes like face cream.

Though we understand that after reading this you may want to stick to the real stuff, you can order safe-sex food products by calling Party Gals at 1-800-621-4841, Doc Johnson Enterprises at 1-800-423-3650 or Kingman Industries at 1-800-255-2441.

to cook together, but it's not good if it turns into a power struggle. "The man might stand there and tell the woman how to chop onions a certain way. She's going to feel offended and criticized," Dr. Virtue says. "If he's really into how onions should be chopped, he should do that."

Maximum Mental Performance

Eating to Boost Your Brainpower

Not even a free month's worth of Twinkies could have convinced any self-respecting seventh grader to trade places with Poindexter. Remember that lanky, pale-faced kid with the supermemory calculator whose right arm hovered over his head throughout class? The one whose mouth seemed to constantly utter, "Oooh, oooh, I know that one." That little brainiac geek was most uncool.

But now we're grown-ups. Poindexter probably owns a computer chip manufacturing company, drives a Lexus and dates a supermodel. And you're not too cool to offer him a month's supply of Twinkies in exchange for his secrets of brainiac success.

Save your Twinkies. We'll give you his secrets for free.

Brain Food

As we age, it gets harder and harder to learn new tricks. Our ability to pick up and remember new information starts slowing down as early as our twenties and continues to gradually decline over the course of our lifetime. "The slowing in memory is tied to the biological deterioration of the nervous system," says Michael Pressley, Ph.D., professor of educational psychology and statis-

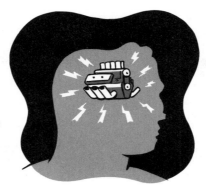

tics at the State University of New York at Albany. "You function more slowly as you get older."

But here are some foods researchers think just might help keep our brains in fine form well into old age.

Sprinkle on lecithin. Our brains have a neurotransmitter called acetycholine that helps us remember stuff. Throughout life, our brains make that memory transmitter from the enzyme choline, which is naturally available in the body. Problem is, doctors think our bodies may make less choline as we age. Lecithin is one of the few things we can eat that can help the body secrete more choline.

In one study 41 people ages 50 to 80 who ate two tablespoons (13.5 grams) of lecithin a day forgot fewer names and misplaced fewer things. The top lecithin food sources are liver, egg yolks and peanuts. Unfortunately, all of those foods also are high in fat and cholesterol. And those are among the first foods that people cut out as they become more health-conscious. Lecithin also is plentiful in soybean products, but let's face it—given a choice between soyburgers or liver, most guys would rather eat, well, almost anything else.

There is a fairly simple solution: Instead of eating high-fat foods or choking down soyburgers, you can buy lecithin in granulated form and sprinkle it on cereal, according to Steven Zeisel, M.D., Ph.D., chairman of the nutrition department at the University of North Carolina at Chapel Hill.

Don't be a moron, eat boron. Boron, found in fruits, nuts and vegetables, is not considered an essential nutrient, but researchers have found that it may help boost brainpower. One study found that people who ate 3.25 milligrams of the micronutrient a day—roughly three-quarters of a cup of peanuts—scored better on manual dexterity, eye-hand coordination, attention, memory and perception tests than those who didn't.

Think before you drink. You've heard this before: Alcohol kills brain cells. It's true. Researchers studying corpses have found that brains of alcohol abusers weigh less than brains of nonalcoholics. Years of excessive drinking leaves brains with less white matter and cerebral cells. You only need to drink a couple of beers a day over a period of years to reduce your intelligence and memory.

Eat breakfast. Brains need fuel to think. You might be able to skip breakfast and cruise through the morning, but you're in for a huge crash in the afternoon, says Elizabeth Somer, R.D., author of *Food and Mood.*

Don't stuff yourself. When you pig out during any meal, you're telling your brain to take a nap. The blood heads to your stomach and away from your head. If you eat a lot of fat, you're really in for a snooze. The fat interferes with the ability of red blood cells to carry oxygen to your brain and tissues, and that cuts down on your brain's oxygen supply. To keep your brain awake, Somer suggests eating every three to four hours. That way, you'll supply constant fuel to your brain and muscles and cut down the odds of overeating.

Snack in the afternoon. Here's one you should like. A study conducted at Tufts University in Medford, Massachusetts, found that eating in midafternoon—whether it's yogurt or a chocolate candy bar—increased students' memory and attention skills. Students who only drank diet soda may have quenched their thirst but not their thirst for knowledge. Before you reach for that candy bar, though, you should know that students who ate the yogurt did even better than those who had the sugar snack. (You didn't really expect scientists to tell you to scarf down candy bars, did you?)

Do a slow burn on sugar. It's true. Sugar gives you a quick boost, but it also dumps directly into your bloodstream. The sudden increase in blood sugar causes your body to produce insulin, which makes your blood sugar drop. The result: You get tired.

Instead of candy bars, you would do better to eat fruit. It has sugar in it, known as fructose, but it's a different kind of sugar. The body has to first break down fructose before it can burn it for energy. The sugar is released into the blood slowly, more evenly and over a longer time, says James M. Rippe, M.D., associate professor of medicine and director of the Center for Clinical and Lifestyle Research at Tufts University Medical School in Shrewsbury, Massachusetts.

Take a coffee break. Caffeine can be a mind-accelerating mood booster when taken in moderation at the right time, says Judith Wurtman, Ph.D., a nutrition research scientist in the Department of Brain and Cognitive Sciences at Massachusetts Institute of Technology in Cambridge, in her book, *Managing Your Mind and Mood through Food.* "There is this tremendous genetic variability among people about how sensitive they are to caffeine," Dr. Rippe says. "They have to find out what amount of coffee fits with who they are genetically."

Hold your intake to no more than three five-ounce cups of java a day. If you drink more, it's likely the coffee will actually make you more tired than alert in the long run, Somer says. And space it out. Your body is most sensitive to caffeine after it hasn't had it in a while, says Dr. Wurtman. To start your day in top mental form, she recommends drinking a cup or two of caffeinated coffee soon after getting up in the morning. A cup in midafternoon will also reawaken your brain and help power your mind for another six hours or so.

Look to the sea. You might have heard that fish is brain food. And that's somewhat true. Some fish have nutrients that are good for your brain. Tuna has important B vitamins, which can help improve your cognitive skills and memory. And oysters and herring are packed with zinc, which also can help prevent memory loss.

Beating Stress

*Staying in the Kitchen
When the Heat's On*

Back in our Neanderthal days, stress meant a huge, snarly, salivating, sharp-toothed, hungry tiger. Our glands secreted chemicals that dilated our pupils, flared our nostrils, tensed our muscles and quickened our breath and pulse. We were ready to either club the beast on the head or run for the cave.

Today stress often comes in the form of a fat, snarly, spits-when-he-talks, sharp-tongued, power-hungry boss. He produces the same result as the tiger. But we can't stand our ground (we'd get fired) and we can't run (we'd get fired), so we're constantly on alert. And that makes us more susceptible to heart disease, ulcers, asthma and cancer.

Stress takes a toll on our bodies. It reduces our absorption and increases our excretion of nutrients. Because we're losing nutrients, we especially need to eat well when stressed out. Unfortunately, it's when we eat our worst.

Instead of eating cereal for breakfast, we grab doughnuts on the way to work. Instead of eating a healthful lunch, we get french fries and a burger on the run at a fast-food joint. Or we skip it altogether. Instead of eating a normal dinner, we snack on potato chips.

"The biggest problem people get into when they are busy is that they violate normal nutrition," says Tufts University's Dr. James M. Rippe. "It's not that there's some magic food that they can eat, it's that they should try not to deviate from eating normal meals."

While interviewing corporate executives for his book, *Fit for Success*, Dr. Rippe found that "the biggest problem

they had when they were coming through the ranks is that they would work odd hours. They wouldn't eat all day, then they would grab a pizza on the way home."

Stress-Blasting Strategies

Here are some ways to help you conquer stress.

Arm yourself. Sometimes you just know when it's going to be bad. Maybe you have a proposal up for review. Or you have a job interview. Then again, sometimes you go in for an easy day but walk into a madhouse instead. You need to be prepared. That means following a healthy diet all the time.

"You want to go into an expected stressful situation well-armed," says registered dietitian Elizabeth Somer. "To try to backtrack and start eating well when you're more than likely going to be eating terribly isn't very likely. What you want to do is boost up your nutrient stores. Have a well-stocked antioxidant system and strong immune system based on a good intake of all the vitamins and minerals. Then when stress hits you from the backside, you're going into it fully armed."

Plan ahead. Bring healthy snacks along to work. That way, when you get the stress munchies, you won't have to rely on the vending machines. "Bring some apples and things rather than candy bars," suggests Dr. Rippe.

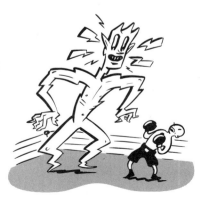

Get some help. When Dr. Rippe asked busy executives how they manage to eat nutritionally during times of stress, the most successful ones had someone by their side. If you can get someone (hint: wife or girlfriend) to pack some turkey sandwiches and carrot sticks for you on the really busy days, you'll have an easier time eating well. Just make sure you return the favor.

Carbo-load to calm down.

Sometimes when we're stressed out, it's too obvious. We sweat. Our hands shake. Our tongues get parched. When you really just need to calm down, think carbohydrate. Eating carbohydrates makes our brains produce the calming chemical serotonin. So if stress is getting the best of your nerves, find a quiet place and have a low-fat carbohydrate snack. Snacks that involve crunching or sucking are especially soothing. Think popcorn, rice cakes, cereal, lollipops, frozen pops and sour balls.

You can even precalm yourself. Let's say you're about to go into a grueling meeting. Eat some carbohydrates about a half-hour before, says Massachusetts Institute of Technology's Dr. Judith Wurtman. You'll need about 1½ ounces of carbohydrates—two cups of Cheerios—for the calming effect to take place, Dr. Wurtman says.

Water your brain.

Maybe you're not the type who gets those embarrassing football-shaped sweat marks under your arms, but that doesn't mean you're not sweating. The average office worker loses ten cups of fluid a day. And your brain is the first organ affected by dehydration, says Paul J. Rosch, M.D., president of the American Institute of Stress and clinical professor of medicine and psychiatry at New York Medical College in Yonkers.

Oftentimes, your body needs water well before your tongue starts telling you to get a drink. So if you're feeling tired, it might be because you're dehydrated, Dr. Rosch says. Caffeinated beverages rob more water from your body than they replace. For every cup of coffee, you should drink two glasses of water.

Eat more fiber.

Stress plays havoc with our digestive systems. Some researchers advise that when you are under stress, you should eat at least five servings of fiber-rich fruits and vegetables, six servings of 100 percent whole-grain breads and cereals and a serving of cooked

---

Sleeping through Stress

Can't sleep because of that presentation you have to make in the morning? A low-fat, low-calorie carbohydrate snack should help put you out, says Massachusetts Institute of Technology's Dr. Judith Wurtman. According to Dr. Wurtman, here are some snacks that should work as sleeping pills.

- 1½ cups of breakfast cereal without milk
- 1½ ounces of caramel-coated popcorn
- Three fig bars
- Six ginger snaps
- One cinnamon raisin English muffin
- One ⅝-ounce package of cinnamon spice instant oatmeal
- One toaster-size frozen waffle with one tablespoon of maple syrup

---

dried peas or beans to keep your digestion running smoothly. But Dr. Rosch cautions that even though eating more fiber and fruit can improve general health, some people with irritable bowel syndrome may not benefit from adding more fiber to their diets.

Take a multivitamin.

When the pressure's on, your nutritional requirements may increase. If, despite your best intentions, you still don't eat right, multivitamin tablets are there as a backup. Look for one that gives you 100 percent of the Recommended Dietary Allowance for all vitamins and minerals, especially the B vitamins, calcium, magnesium, chromium, copper, iron, manganese, molybdenum, selenium and zinc.

Take a walk.

Instead of reaching for a cigarette, candy bar or soda, take a walk. "For people who are highly anxious, simply taking a walk will give them an immediate and significant reduction in stress," Dr. Rippe says. "Most people feel the benefit they're getting from walking is not just the exercise but also the time out. You're getting away from the stressful environment."

Excelling at Sports

How to Eat to Compete

Milo of Croton was one amazing dude. In the sixth century B.C. the six-time Greek Olympic wrestling champion was a master of strength, balance and control. He could hold a pomegranate so tightly no one could extricate it from his hand, yet so gently he squeezed no juice from the orange-size berry. He could wrap cord around his forehead and slice it in half by furrowing his brow. And he could fend off attackers while balancing on an oiled disk.

Milo also ate like a pig. A typical Milo meal included seven pounds of meat and seven pounds of bread. Had the Greek Olympic committee hired a registered dietitian for Milo, it's entirely possible he would have found even more amazing feats up his toga.

The dietitian would have told Milo to eat a pound more of bread and a pound less of meat. Here's why. Athletes get energy from a substance called glycogen that is stored in muscles and the liver. When Milo threw other wrestlers to the ground, broke cords with his head and performed other feats, he burned glycogen. But when he ate his seven pounds of bread, he replenished only some of it.

Bread is a carbohydrate, and any excess carbohydrate that the body doesn't use as fuel gets stored in the liver and muscles as glycogen. A normal guy needs carbohydrates to make up between 60 and 65 percent of his diet. An endurance athlete, like Milo, who trains to exhaustion daily, needs more like 65 to 70 percent to keep the muscles fueled. So if Milo ate eight pounds of bread and cut back to six pounds of meat, he might have won the pentathlon as well as balanced a statue on his pinkie.

Okay, so it's an extreme example. To be a great athlete, you don't need to eat as much as Milo. You just need to get the proportion right. Bread, rice, potatoes and other carbohydrates should be the major part of your diet and meat and fat the lesser part, says Brenda Gross, R.D., a nutritionist at the Emory Clinic Sports Medicine Center in Decatur, Georgia.

Time to Fuel Up

Choosing the right fuel is only half the battle. You also have to know how to use it at the right time. After all, you could select the highest grade of premium gasoline for your car, but it wouldn't do a bit of good if you wait until you're out of gas to fill your tank. The same goes for your body. Here are some strategies to help you avoid running on empty.

Run and eat. The best time to eat is right after your workout. "That's when your muscles are most receptive to storing carbohydrates. And the muscles are ready to be repaired if you take in a little protein," says Gross.

Try to fit in a carbohydrate snack within a half-hour after working out. Then, within three hours, have a high-carbohydrate meal—potatoes, rice, bread, vegetables or pasta. "That will ensure your muscles are replenished," Gross says. "It's really important for people who work out every day, because they are putting a toll on their bodies."

Eat early. Two hours before working out, fuel up with 200 to 500 calories, mostly from complex carbohydrates. Good foods include cereal, juice and toast because they are easily digested. Do not eat within 45 minutes of working out, says Gross. The carbohydrates could trick your body into overproducing insulin, and you're more sensitive to insulin when exercising. It will make you exhausted, not energized. Also, during exercise, blood is diverted from the stomach to the muscles. If you eat too soon before exercise, the food will remain in your stomach and cause intestinal and stomach upset.

Refuel to fight fatigue. We know we just told you not to eat right before working out, but you can eat during a workout. Eating a piece of fruit or an energy bar during events that last longer than 90 minutes can delay fatigue, says Gross.

Don't gas up. During pre-exercise meals, avoid foods that may cause flatulence and foods that digest slowly. They'll mess up your workout. Foods to avoid include high-fiber, high-carbohydrate ones such as beans, brussels sprouts, brans, onions and peas.

Drink ahead. When competing, have about two cups of a sports beverage about ten minutes before an endurance event to give your muscles some extra fuel, says Gross. The beverage will be able to move out of your stomach faster than solid food.

Eat what you know. The day of competition or an important workout isn't the time for culinary experimentation. If you haven't eaten a certain food before, don't add it to your diet before a training session, Gross says. You don't want to discover that your stomach doesn't digest tuna that well while you're trying to set a personal record in the 5-K.

Quench That Thirst

During a hard workout you can lose between six and eight pounds of sweat an hour.

Power in a Bar?

Just in case you believe everything you see on TV, we have some news for you. Know all those energy bars? They won't turn you into a superathlete. And you should never eat them before a workout.

"During exercise, the blood is carried away from the digestive system and out to the extremities where you're working the muscles," says nutritionist Brenda Gross. "So digestion pretty much comes to a halt during exercise. That's why you don't want to eat just before exercise, because that food is just going to sit there in your stomach the whole time. I recommend fruit over a power bar because fruit will leave the stomach a little bit faster."

But energy bars are good for something: convenience. Triathletes and marathon runners who need to eat during an event can easily stash a power bar somewhere on their bodies. And they easily fit in backpacks for mountain climbers.

Plus, they can be a good postevent snack as long as they are loaded with carbohydrates.

What are the best power bars? You're looking for something high in calories and high in carbohydrates, with some protein, vitamins and minerals. Read the wrapper. Some "power bars" are really candy bars with fancy packaging. Look for bars with less than 30 percent fat and more than 50 percent carbohydrate.

Dehydration drains muscle strength, saps endurance and hampers coordination. It also increases the chances of cramping, heat exhaustion and heatstroke.

You can head off dehydration by drinking at least two cups of liquid two hours before working out. Then have another two cups 15 to 20 minutes before your workout.

Also, drink during your workout.

Ideally, you should try to drink enough water before and during exercise that you won't lose much water weight. But you still should weigh yourself before and after exercise to find out how much you lost, says Gross. And replace each lost pound with 16 ounces of fluid.

For most people, water is the best choice. Endurance athletes, though, should use sports drinks during exercise because the glucose in the beverage can give muscles extra fuel. "If your sport lasts longer than 90 minutes, that's when the sports drinks are more beneficial, because that helps maintain your blood sugar," Gross says. "For sports under 90 minutes, water is just as effective."

Endurance athletes also can use sports drinks like multivitamins. Have one a day. "If you are going to lose more than four pounds of sweat on any occasion, then a sports drink is probably a good idea to add to your daily diet to help replenish you from one day to the next," says Bryant Stamford, Ph.D., director of the Health Promotion and Wellness Center and professor at the University of Louisville.

Here's how to pick a winning sports drink.

Get the right mix. Don't bother searching for a drink packed with minerals and other stuff hyped by commercials. Your diet will replenish all of them. What you want is glucose—fuel. But you don't want too much of it. Don't buy anything with more than 8 percent glucose, fructose or any other sugar. "When you get more than 8 percent glucose in it, it takes longer to empty the stomach, so it's not getting out to the muscles as quickly," Gross says.

Go for taste. This is common sense.

Muscle Meals

If you want to beef up your biceps, you don't need to chow down on steak.

It's true, bodybuilders do need a bit more protein than the average Joe. But the thing is, they're already getting it. "Most people take in a lot more protein than they already need," says nutritionist Brenda Gross. "All the protein most people need is in a couple of glasses of milk or four ounces of meat."

Your body normally needs about .01 ounces per pound of body weight daily. Weight lifters need about .02 ounces per pound of body weight. Most men eat twice as much—more than 3.5 ounces. Instead of adding protein, make the protein you do eat lean. Go for fish, skinless chicken, lean beef or turkey.

Like other athletes, what you'll probably need more of is carbohydrates. Your body can then burn the carbohydrates for fuel and use your protein to build muscle.

Male athletes should shoot for 20 to 25 servings of high-carbohydrate foods a day, says Gross. That's not as hard as it sounds. The average bowl of Shredded Wheat cereal with a banana counts as 5 servings. Two sandwiches (with four slices of bread) make 4 more. A pasta salad and

You want a drink that you like. That way you'll drink it, and you won't get dehydrated.

Powder Power

In any health food store you'll find an array of items that are supposed to boost your athletic prowess. Few are medically proven. Here's a look at the pros and cons of a few common performance aids.

• Creatine. Naturally found in meat and

baked potato for dinner would add about 9 more. And snacking on bagels and muffins in the morning and afternoon would bring you to 20.

Here are some other muscle-building techniques to keep in mind.

Eat up. It takes 2,500 extra calories to build a pound of muscle. For every hour you lift you need 300 to 500 additional calories, says Gross. Good high-carbohydrate, low-fat, 500-calorie snacks include a cup of cereal with skim milk; a banana and four tablespoons of raisins; a cup of low-fat yogurt and six fig bars; and a bagel, a pint of grape juice and an apple.

Feast on fruit. You need calories to gain weight, and vegetables hardly have any. So eat fruit. One 60-calorie serving—the equivalent of about one orange—more than doubles what you would get from a vegetable. But don't forget your vegetables for vitamins, minerals and fiber, adds Gross.

Drink all day. Drink a glass of water every hour during the days you train. Your muscles need it. Water makes up 69 to 75 percent of muscle fiber and is used for everything from contraction to cooling, says Gross.

sylvania State University in University Park, warns that long-term intake has not been studied, so the potential consequences of regular intake are not known. Those who took the supplements for studies had between 20 and 30 grams over five days.

• Glycerol. After long exercise the body begins to dehydrate. Water helps, but you usually can't offset how much you sweat. Glycerol is a natural substance that has been shown to enhance the body's ability to retain water, allowing longer, better exercise. When glycerol is taken in, it slows your output of urine, says Paul Montner, M.D., of the University of New Mexico in Albuquerque, so more water is available during endurance sports when fluids are at a premium. It has some possible side effects: headache and stomachache. Glycerol is still considered experimental by most researchers, and Dr. Montner warns that you shouldn't try it without medical supervision.

• Multivitamin/mineral supplements. In laboratory and field tests multivitamin and mineral supplements have not been found to improve performance. But you may want to take a daily multivitamin just to offset nutrient loss that occurs during exercise, says Gross. It will come in handy on those days when you just don't get in all of your food groups. Take the tablet with food. It increases your chances that the nutrients will be absorbed into your system.

• Salt tablets. Once a staple in high school locker rooms, it's now on the must-avoid list, says Gross. Water, high-nutrient food and occasional salted snacks will replace whatever salt you lose during exercise. Even if you lost nine pounds of sweat during exercise, you would only lose about 5 to 7 percent of your body's salt content.

fish, creatine supplements may enhance stamina. In some studies, volunteers could cycle and sprint with less fatigue when they were taking creatine supplements. It may work by helping the muscles use adenosine triphosphate, the primary fuel for cells. Using that fuel more efficiently speeds up the muscle recovery rate and delays fatigue. Creatine supplements are available in health food stores, but Wayne W. Campbell, Ph.D., an applied physiologist at the Noll Physiological Research Center at Penn-

Hot and Cold Weather

Setting Your Own Climate Control

Researchers at Johns Hopkins University in Baltimore have studied our weather-related eating habits for years. And they have us pretty well figured out. In the summer when our bodies have switched to a low-calorie burning mode, we eat lots of raw vegetables, drink plenty of fluids and chow on carbohydrates and sweets.

In the winter we switch to fat and protein. We eat a lot more and a lot more often.

And we get fat.

Some of us lose it. Some of us don't. We just gain more weight the next winter and keep getting more and more rotund.

"We find appetites usually increase in winter for psychological and physiological reasons," says Maria Simonson, Sc.D., Ph.D., director of the Health, Weight and Stress Clinic at Johns Hopkins Medical Institutions in Baltimore. "You're going to eat more even if you're snugly inside, because food has the psychological effect of making us feel more secure and protected from the bad weather outside. That's why when you're inside in the winter, you will have a tendency to nibble. It feels cozier if you have a cup of hot chocolate and something to nibble on."

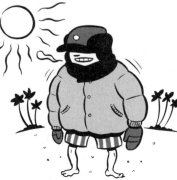

In the Summertime

If you don't pay attention, the weather will control your diet. If you do pay attention, you can't control the weather, but you can control your diet. Here are a few ways to outsmart Mother Nature when the heat is on.

Drink water. You know this. But we're going to tell you again because—if you're like most of us—you don't do it. Even though it's common sense, few of us drink enough water. It's especially important in the summer when you are losing a lot of fluid by sweating. And sweating, after all, is your body's odoriferous, but effective, cooling system. Make sure to drink about ten eight-ounce glasses of liquid a day, says Neva Cochran, R.D., a private nutrition consultant and a spokesperson for the American Dietetic Association in Dallas.

Go slow on the booze. In The Kinks' classic summertime song, "Sunny Afternoon," lead singer Ray Davies dispenses some sound health advice: "Now I'm sittin' here, sippin' at my ice cold beer, lazing on a sunny afternoon." The key word is sipping. If nothing tastes as good as an ice cold beer on a hot summer day, then by all means grab one and head for the hammock. But if you're having more than one, look out. The heat increases the effect of alcohol on the brain.

Let's say five drinks makes you start eyeing lampshades as headgear in normal weather. When it's hot, expect to start acting stupid after only three drinks, Dr. Simonson says. And you have more to worry about than being scared to show your face the next day.

Booze also dehydrates you at a time when you're losing more water to sweat.

Don't scream for ice cream. Drinking really cold drinks or eating something cold such as ice cream might make you feel cooler for about 15 minutes, but they won't cool your body. Body heat is controlled by calories. So when you have a cold, high-calorie snack such as a milk shake or ice cream, you're going to make yourself hotter.

"The calories are what determines your coolness or your warmth. Ice cream will give you more body heat than the warmth that lasts 10 or 15 minutes from a hot bowl of soup because the calories are higher," Dr. Simonson says.

Avoid dressing up. Many people like to drink a lot of fruit juice and eat cold-cut salads with oily dressings in the summer. It just seems like light eating, but it's not. Oily dressings are packed with fat calories, and many fruit drinks are loaded with sugar calories.

Weathering Winter

There's something to be said for foraging outside in the Arctic region: food. You can eat and eat and eat without gaining weight. That's because it's so cold your body needs about 7,000 calories a day just to keep you warm.

Theoretically, winter is the best time to lose weight. Realistically, however, most of us gain 7.43 pounds between October and April.

What's going on here? For one, we usually stay in the heated indoors during the winter. So we're not cold. And even though we do need extra calories, we tend to eat much more than we need. Here are some ways to keep off winter weight gain and stay warm.

Don't be fooled. You already learned that ice cream won't make you cold, so now it's time to learn that soup won't make you hot. Sure it will warm the area around your stomach and intestines for about 15 minutes, but it will also make the blood vessels in your skin dilate. You'll feel warmer, but you're really losing heat.

Switch to snacking. Instead of eating three winter meals a day, have five. The constant calories will make you feel warmer, and spreading them out will help you control your weight as long as the portions are smaller. "If you have a habit of eating more and more frequent meals, less of what you eat

will turn to fat," Dr. Simonson says.

Stay active. If you keep activity up in winter, you will be able to keep weight down. "It requires a lot more energy and more effort to generate body heat. Besides, you wear more clothes in winter and that increases your energy expenditure," Dr. Simonson says.

Cut the fat. You're going to crave fat and protein in the winter. It's okay to go with the protein. It will help you stay warm. But forget the fat. Go for lean meats, poultry and fish to satisfy your cravings, says Dr. Simonson.

Remove temptation. When you're cooped up in the house, you might linger around the kitchen table. Instead of letting snack cakes, cheese curls and potato chips stare you in the face, keep them locked up in a dark cupboard. Or don't buy them until the spring thaw. Instead, make sure more nutritious, lower-fat items such as grapes and oranges are within reach, suggests Dr. Simonson.

Drink up. Instead of eating every time you feel the urge to snack, have something to drink. Liquids move to your intestines faster than solid food and they make you feel fuller sooner. Liquid intake is important in the winter because your body can easily become dehydrated as it works extra hard to moisten and warm the cold air you inhale, says Cochran.

Pretend it's summer. You're better off sticking to a lighter, summer-style eating habit during the winter. Have soup and salad nights. Make it a hearty soup like chicken or vegetable or bean. They take longer to eat, says Dr. Simonson, so your brain has a chance to register that your stomach is full before you overeat.

Spice it up. Spicy foods can help cut calories because you eat less of them. They also make you feel warm, says Dr. Simonson.

Play it safe. There's nothing like a hot toddy on a cold day, but drinking booze during cold weather can be deceiving. It makes you feel warm, yet it makes blood vessels near the skin's surface dilate, actually causing heat loss.

Preventing Disease

Eat to Beat the Reaper

What kind of stakes do you like to gamble for? Maybe you don't mind plunking down a buck for a lottery ticket, even knowing that your chances of winning the jackpot are practically zip. You might happily wager much more on a longshot horse or a handful of poker cards.

But how comfortable are you with betting your life? Suppose you found out that you could reduce—by 40 percent—the odds of having your life cut short by colon cancer? That's a no-brainer—you'd take the safe route. And that protection is yours when you adopt a diet high in grains and vegetables.

Suppose you learned that you could shave your risk of heart disease 12 percent by lowering your cholesterol level just 10 percent? If you're starting with a cholesterol count of 240, that's the protection you'll gain. (It's best to be under 200.)

Your Weapons against Disease

More than a million men die in the United States each year. Three-quarters of those deaths involve diseases directly related to nutrition—heart disease, cancer, stroke and diabetes. The nutrition-and-disease connection is a hot area of scientific research, and a lot is still unknown about how food protects your body. But

researchers agree that nutrition influences degenerative diseases in these ways.

- Eating poorly can make a disease develop more rapidly.
- Healthful eating can prevent disease.
- Healthful eating can ease the effect of degenerative diseases that you do get.

Exactly how these wonders occur is the subject of fervent debate. The benefits of fiber, minerals and vitamins—especially the cancer-fighting antioxidants—are probably familiar to you by now. But researchers are making almost daily revelations about other protective plant chemicals that carry alien names like flavonoids, indoles and lignans. Hundreds of these substances are yet to be thoroughly analyzed for how they accomplish their good deeds. But there's no need to sit back on your haunches. Scientists state unequivocally that these basic practices will bolster you against some of the country's biggest killer diseases.

- Eating lots of different kinds of foods.
- Controlling your weight by balancing the amount of food you eat with exercise.
- Eating lots of complex carbohydrates.
- Limiting your consumption of fat, cholesterol, sugar, salt and alcohol.

Keeping Your Arteries Free and Clear

Heart attack and stroke are the number one and number three killers of men in the United States. But lifestyle factors that you control have a lot to do with whether you will be felled by these maladies.

The causes of heart attack and stroke are very similar. Fatty deposits cling to the inner walls of your arteries, a condition called atherosclerosis. As these deposits grow and harden, the arteries narrow and become less flexible. This drives up your

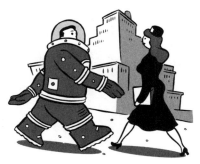

blood pressure. Ultimately, less blood flows through the kidneys, and they respond by raising the blood pressure even more, which puts stress on the heart. Unfortunately, high blood pressure damages those rigid arteries, creating spots where plaque is even more likely to build up. Yes, you read right: Arterial plaque and high blood pressure aggravate each other, creating a nasty spiral.

Blood clots can form at the site of plaque buildup. If a clot breaks free of the artery wall, it follows the bloodstream until it lodges in a passage that's too narrow. Deprived of blood, the tissue beyond that passage quickly dies. If that tissue happens to be the heart, you've had a heart attack. If the tissue happens to be the brain, that's a stroke.

How do you lower your risk of a heart attack or stroke? You can influence three of the prime risk factors with the way you eat.

Get the count down. Doctors say it's best to keep your cholesterol count under 200. The keys, once again, are a low-fat diet and exercise. This means eating plenty of plant food. Use low-fat or nonfat dairy products and limit your consumption of eggs, cheese and meat.

To reaffirm the effect of diet on cholesterol, researchers at the University of Kentucky in Lexington compared men's and women's cholesterol readings during eight weeks of an American Heart Association diet. The diet called for 30 percent of their calories to come from fat, 50 to 60 percent from carbohydrates and 10 to 20 percent from protein.

The researchers found the diet to be equally effective for men and women. The 99 men lowered their readings by an average of 7.2 percent, while the 63 women lowered their cholesterol an average of 9.2 percent. And those who started with the highest cholesterol readings showed the most dramatic improvement.

Here, Phyto

Maybe you know your vitamins and minerals. But phytochemicals are a class of substances that even researchers don't have a handle on yet. They're not essential chemicals, meaning you could live without them (unlike vitamins and many minerals). But many are thought to have disease-fighting qualities. While there are hundreds of phytochemicals, only a few have been studied extensively. Here's a sampling.

- **Flavonoids.** These chemicals are found in lots of fruits, vegetables and in wine. They're thought to reduce cancer risk either by preventing carcinogens from getting into cells, preventing cancerous changes in cells or interfering with harmful hormone processes.

- **Indoles and isothiocyanates.** These chemicals put the zing in the taste of cruciferous vegetables (broccoli, brussels sprouts, cabbage, cauliflower and the like). They're thought to stop carcinogens from reaching cells, and isothiocyanates may also interfere with tumor growth.

- **Isoflavones.** These guys make a heavy showing in soybeans and soy products, which may explain why Asian men have a lower prostate cancer rate. Isoflavones are thought to work as antioxidants, to block cancer-causing substances or to suppress tumors.

- **Lignans.** Linseeds, the seeds from flax, are particularly heavy in lignans. They're thought to be an antioxidant and may block or suppress malignant changes in cells.

- **Organosulfur compounds.** Found in garlic, onions, leeks and shallots. These chemicals may block or suppress tumor growth.

Get your weight down. If you're overweight, consider this: For every 10 percent reduction in weight, you'll gain a 20 percent reduction in the risk of cardiovascular disease. So follow a low-fat diet (lots of rice, pasta, beans, fruits, vegetables, fish and chicken) and exercise.

"We've become a sedentary population. That means less energy expenditure. We've also adopted a relatively high-fat diet. Since fat contains concentrated calories, that can mean more calories in your diet. The combination of less energy output and more caloric input leads to weight gain," says Christopher Gardner, Ph.D., a research fellow at the Stanford Center for Research in Disease Prevention. "It's easier to lose weight—or prevent gaining weight—with a low-fat diet. Losing weight, regardless of whether you do it through exercise or diet or a combination, can have a dramatic and beneficial impact on cholesterol and triglyceride levels in the blood."

Take the pressure off. To control your blood pressure, once again you need to keep your weight down and exercise. Follow a low-fat, high-fiber diet, meaning loads of whole grains, beans, vegetables and fruits. Make sure you get foods that are high in potassium (cauliflower, spinach, potatoes, orange juice), calcium (nonfat yogurt, skim milk, sardines) and magnesium (leafy green vegetables, seafood, dairy products). Limit your consumption of sodium and alcohol.

Your Shield against Cancer

Cancer is a disease in which cells of the body are altered, allowing them to multiply out of control. The food you eat can intervene in this process. Since cancer is the second-leading cause of death of American men, you'll want to under- stand how this works. First consider the stages of cancer development.

- The body is exposed to a cancer-causing chemical called a carcinogen.
- The carcinogen affects the cell membrane and can enter the cell.
- The carcinogen can also alter the cell's DNA.
- Other factors in the body encourage development of the cancer, and the cells multiply.
- A mass of cells called a tumor forms, interfering with normal body functions.

Now, one obvious strategy in preventing cancer is to avoid the carcinogens that get the process rolling in the first place. That's why you should avoid smoking, as well as water and air pollution. In the diet, limit your consumption of foods preserved by salt, smoke and nitrites.

You can also limit your risk of cancer by eating less of the foods that "promote" tumor growth—that is, the foods that encourage development of cancerous cells once you've been exposed to a carcinogen. Fat is a major culprit in this respect. Scientists believe a high-fat diet may promote cancer growth in a number of ways: by prompting hormone secretions that aid cancer; by prompting bile secretions into the intestine, where it may be converted into cancer-causing compounds; and by weakening cell membranes against cancer-causing agents. Fat may also weaken the immune system.

So while there's no indication that fat is the original cause of tumors, "there's a lot of information on fat promoting tumor growth," says Michael J. González, D.Sc., Ph.D., assistant professor of nutritional biochemistry and advanced nutrition at the University of Puerto Rico Medical Sciences Campus School of Public Health in San Juan. "Once the tumor is there, fat will aid its growth."

Not all fat is equally harmful in this respect. Linoleic acid, the fat found in vegetable oils, is a prime suspect in the promotion of cancer. Monounsaturates (olive and canola oil) and omega-3 fatty acids (fish oil), however, don't seem to have any such effect.

Many plant foods offer protection from

cancer. Studies show that fiber (found in whole grains, beans, fruits and vegetables) helps you resist colon cancer, apparently by sweeping bile out of the intestine before harmful chemicals can have any effect. And research confirms that people who eat lots of fruits and vegetables—particularly the green, yellow and orange ones—are less likely to get a variety of cancers, including mouth, throat, stomach, bladder, breast and prostate cancer. Scientists theorize that antioxidants found in fruits and vegetables, like beta-carotene and vitamins C and E, disarm harmful molecules in the body called free radicals.

But the secret to protective nutrition is not to pounce upon, say, sweet potatoes and scarf them down relentlessly. There are many other vitamins, minerals and food chemicals that are thought to inhibit cancer, too. They're undergoing intense study—vitamins B_6 and B_{12}, folate, pantothenic acid, zinc, selenium and more. You won't find all of the protective chemicals in any one food. Besides, some of these substances may protect you not by working alone but in concert with chemicals from other plants. Furthermore, a repetitive diet is a risky one. Eating a broad variety of foods dilutes the effect of any harmful substances you may consume.

Bottom line: Mom was right. Eat your vegetables, and lots of 'em.

Chase Away the Blood Sugar Blues

In the hierarchy of killer diseases, diabetes only ranks number seven among American males. But we're still talking about 21,000 men killed each year, so it's nothing to sneeze at. Besides, it's another disease with

---

The Cancer Connection

Here are dietary factors that affect various specific cancers.

- **Esophagus. Risk factors: High alcohol and tobacco use (particularly in combination); low vitamin and mineral intake. Protective factor: Daily variety of fruits and vegetables.**

- **Stomach. Risk factor: High intake of food preserved in salt. Protective factor: High consumption of fruits and vegetables.**

- **Colon. Risk factors: High intake of fat and alcohol. Protective factor: High intake of vegetables.**

- **Pancreas and lung. Risk factor: Smoking. Protective factor: Green and yellow vegetables.**

- **Bladder. Risk factor: Smoking. Possible risk factors: Coffee, artificial sweeteners, alcohol. Protective factor: Green and yellow vegetables.**

- **Prostate. Risk factor: High-fat diet. Protective factor: Green and yellow vegetables.**

---

such a heavy dietary connection that you have a substantial amount of control over its effects.

Diabetes is a disease involving a metabolism gone haywire. In the two main forms of the disease, the body is not able to move enough blood sugar out of the blood and into cells where it is needed for energy. In one form, the pancreas loses the ability to produce enough insulin, which is supposed to transfer blood sugar out of the blood. This condition is called insulin-dependent diabetes mellitus, because the patient has to inject insulin now and then to get the job done.

In the second form of diabetes, the insulin is there but it's not effective enough in removing sugar from the blood—a condition called insulin resistance. This variety of the disease, covering 80 percent of all cases, is called non-insulin-dependent diabetes mellitus. It tends to surface later in life, since the ability of the pancreas to produce insulin declines with age. Being overweight also is a factor: The more body fat you have, the higher your insulin resistance. People with this form of diabetes may also need extra insulin if dietary controls are not sufficient.

Without sufficient insulin and with blood sugar soaring, the body enters a complex riot of reactions as it tries to cope with a hampered energy supply system. The patient urinates excessively and dehydrates. The blood's acid-base balance tilts toward acid. Sodium and potassium are flushed from the body, increasing the blood acidity and creating the risk of a coma. (People with non-insulin-dependent diabetes generally do not have the acidity problem since the insulin present in their blood prevents the acid buildup. They do run the risk, however, of a coma brought on by extremely high blood sugar.)

Uncontrolled diabetes can be deadly. Small arteries can be blocked or destroyed, making amputation of feet or legs necessary. Circulation problems may lead to a heart attack or stroke. Other complications can include loss of sight, loss of sensation in the limbs, loss of kidney function and susceptibility to infection.

Don't Wait—Eat Folate

Pssst. Buddy. How would you like to cut your odds of getting coronary artery disease by 10 percent?

Interested? Then help yourself to more pinto and kidney beans, asparagus, brussels sprouts and mustard greens. These foods are full of folate, a B vitamin that has a clear link to lowering the risk of heart disease. Research shows that if people would increase their daily total of this vitamin to 400 micrograms, between 13,500 to 50,000 deaths from coronary artery disease could be prevented each year. That might reduce the risk of artery disease more than 10 percent for men.

You can get your daily dose of 400 micrograms of folic acid from most multivitamins, but by now, you know you probably should be eating more fruits and vegetables anyway.

The only caution regarding supplements: in older people, high amounts of folic acid may mask dangerous deficiencies in vitamin B$_{12}$. So older people should check with their doctors before taking supplements.

The Anti-diabetes Diet

The strategy for preventing diabetes may sound familiar: Eat lots of fiber and complex carbohydrates and limit sugar and fat. Complex carbohydrates do not surge into your bloodstream as quickly as simple sugars, says Benjamin Caballero, M.D., Ph.D., director of the Center for Human Nutrition at Johns Hopkins University in Baltimore. Therefore, they have a leveling effect on blood sugar. "They demand

less insulin," he says, "so your pancreas doesn't have to work as much. They're more efficiently used by the body."

If you already have diabetes, the approach for managing the disease is likely to be similar. The main goal will be to reduce the complications of the disease by controlling blood sugar and blood fats, like cholesterol and triglycerides. But because diabetic conditions are highly individual, you're going to need the assistance of a dietitian or physician.

For overweight men with non-insulin-dependent diabetes, trimming pounds is going to be key. The greater the weight loss, the more improvement in blood sugar control, insulin sensitivity and blood fat levels.

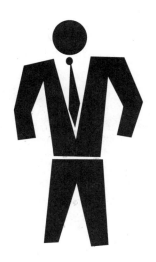

Part Five

Real-Life Scenarios

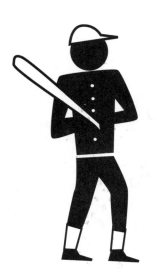

Quest for the Best
They're world-beaters: successful, celebrated and at the top of their games. Over the years, they've learned to eat for pleasure, health and peak performance. Here are their secrets for eating right.

You Can Do It!
These guys are juggling jobs, families and other important factors—just like you. Although they have different stories to tell, they share at least one thing in common: a commitment to eating right. They're food smart—and you can be, too.

Male Makeovers
Eating right can be tough in today's fast-paced world. There are a dizzying array of choices, and it's not always easy to make the correct one. Our experts give their advice on how to be food smart.

Quest for the Best   They're world-beaters: successful, celebrated and at the top of their games. Over the years, they've learned to eat for pleasure, health and peak performance. Here are their secrets for eating right.

Herschel Walker, Professional Football Player

Following His Own Game Plan

When he was a junior in high school, Herschel Walker was already an overachiever. And he was already embarking on his famous one-meal-a-day approach to nutrition.

"I was going to be graduated early, and I had a chance to get out of school around lunchtime," says Walker, now a backfield powerhouse for the New York Giants. "Instead of going to lunch, I would go to work—I was a mechanic's helper. I wanted to get in as many hours as I could before I had to go to practice."

And that's pretty much how Walker eats now, in his midthirties. Oh, there was a time at the University of Georgia when that dinner could consist of Snickers bars, but nowadays he restricts himself to chicken, rice and loads of fruits and vegetables.

"I got to where my body really was not asking for any food," Walker says. "I think as Americans we have a tendency to overeat. We really don't need that much food, and I think I'm living proof of that. You know, I survive and I don't get fatigued. I have a lot of energy and I'm healthy, and so I just do it. I don't make myself eat. I only eat when I want to eat.

"There are some days

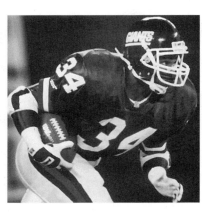

when I might not eat at all. I don't eat a pregame meal, and if we're playing Sunday afternoon, I may not eat that whole day—maybe not until Monday night. It's really according to how I feel."

Making Adjustments

A skimpy diet wouldn't be so surprising if Walker were, say, a geeky video-games champion.

But Walker is a sculpted, 220-pound, six-foot, 29½-inch-waist, athletic perpetual motion machine. He works out a minimum of six hours a day, far longer than he sleeps each night—four hours. (Walker hates to waste time. Any more time in the sack and he goes stir crazy.)

He jogs and sprints eight to ten miles a day off-season and four to six miles in-season—not counting his footwork on the field. He doesn't pump iron but his calisthenics are legendary: as many as 3,000 sit-ups and 1,500 push-ups. All of it, seven days a week.

You could probably feed your body much like he does, he says, if you built up to it very gradually. "I've always said some of the things I do are good for me, but they may not be good for anyone else," he says. "But I think it would work for a lot of people—they'd just have to eat a little bit more than what I eat, maybe a real light breakfast. Some kind of fruit.

"For lunch maybe have some kind of baked or broiled

chicken and a lot of vegetables. And late at night, not eat that much. Have some more fruit or something. That's about it. You need to try to stay away from a lot of red meat."

Don't try to change your diet all at once, he suggests. "The body can adjust to the food that you feed it, or that you're not feeding it, but you have to give it time. If you've had a routine for a long time, changing it means the body will suffer for a little bit. I think some people make the mistake of trying to do something right now. Well, it won't happen right now. Give yourself time. The body will adjust."

Power Eating

Here's what pro football player Herschel Walker eats in a typical day. Yeah, it's not much, but who's going to argue with him?

Breakfast: Nothing

Lunch: Nothing

Dinner: A standard serving of baked or broiled chicken, rice, lots of vegetables, spinach, a little bread, maybe grapes for dessert

Liquids: Mostly water, occasionally fruit juice

A "Boring" Life

Through all of his varied pursuits, from Olympic bobsledding to martial arts to writing poetry to track to ballet, he feeds himself precisely the same. His body appreciates the consistency.

"A lot of people take the body through so many different changes, which I don't think is good," Walker says. "I think the body is the toughest substance in the world, but you can't put it through a lot of different changes. You have to put it in one field and leave it there—give it time to adjust and the body will adjust."

That dovetails with what he admits is a "boring" personal life. He spends a lot of time with his wife, Cindy. He likes movies, writing and working out. He doesn't party. He doesn't go barhopping.

Two things he has no intention of adjusting to are alcohol and junk food. "I never really was around alcohol," he says, "and as I got older, I saw it was not the smart thing to do. I'm not a follower. I don't have to drink to make myself look big or to be one of the boys. I want people to respect me for who I am, and

that's what I try to be. And I try to keep my head about me at all times.

"I don't eat as much junk food either. I eat a lot of vegetables and rice, more than anything. Spinach—something like that. I eat a lot of grapes, maybe, for dessert."

Staying Young

Walker is considered by many to be the best-conditioned athlete in the National Football League. In Walker's profession, however, his co-workers are commonly a decade younger. Crash-test dummies have gentler careers than professional running backs. The sports commentators ooh and ahh at how injury-free Walker's record is, especially for a man his age.

"Age is in the mind," snorts Walker, the 1982 Heisman Trophy winner. "If a person doesn't think or feel old, he's not going to be that way. I feel good. I feel like I can do things and I just do it. I don't sit around thinking about whether I'm not supposed to because of my age. That's irrelevant. If it feels good, do it. Once you start thinking you're too old to do it, that's when your body is going to start getting old."

Jim Palmer, Hall of Fame Pitcher

Touching All of the Nutritional Bases

The first time Hall of Fame pitcher Jim Palmer really ate healthy, it wasn't by choice.

"In 1968 I'd hurt my arm and I was down in Puerto Rico (for rehab)," the former Baltimore Orioles great recalls. "I went from about 210 or 212 pounds to 190, just because I didn't eat as much junk food. Down there, I was eating more rice and bananas and things like that. More native-type food. And I lost 20 pounds."

Today, almost 30 years later, Palmer still tips the scales in the low 190s. "But I know that, within a matter of moments, I could be at 210 by going back to my old eating habits," he says. "Pie à la mode, eating all the things you know are bad for you but that make you feel good for the moment. I think that's where the discipline comes in."

And that discipline has clearly paid off. Jim Palmer, now in his early fifties, is the Dick Clark of the sporting world. He has maintained his trim, athletic build and boyish good looks long after his remarkable 21-year baseball career ended. Between broadcasting stints for network television and local Orioles games and his commercial campaigns for such high-profile clients as The Money Store and Jockey underwear, Palmer is probably on the tube more now than he was in his playing days.

But Palmer didn't cut any Dorian Gray deals or discover the magic fountain of youth, although he does spend part of the year at his winter home in Juno Beach, Florida. "You make lifestyle decisions," he says. "I don't want to live a boring life. But I want to make conscious decisions that are going to be healthier."

A Major-League Change-Up

Growing up as a three-sport schoolboy star, Palmer never worried much about what he ate. As an all-state football, basketball and baseball player in Arizona in the early 1960s, Palmer's basic diet consisted of the same staples as any other all-American boy's: hamburgers and hot dogs.

"I just felt that whatever I ate would be superseded by going to basketball practice, doing my homework and then going for a two-mile run," Palmer says. "I never worried about the nutritional value. I just felt I would be in good shape, regardless of what I ate. That's how naive I was."

Coming out of high school, Palmer rejected a scholarship offer to play basketball for UCLA. (If he had said yes, he would have played with another pretty fair player, a kid named Lew Alcindor—known around the world today as Kareem Abdul-Jabbar.) The 18-year-old Palmer, meanwhile, got a then-whopping $50,000 bonus to sign with the Orioles.

Once in the minor leagues, though, it was a different story. Players got three dollars a day in meal money, and it didn't go very far. "You'd have grilled cheese sandwiches," Palmer recalls. "Then, everybody said you ought to eat wheat bread. So you'd try to eat healthy by having a grilled cheese sandwich that was fried in butter on whole-wheat bread."

When he hit the majors, Palmer quickly

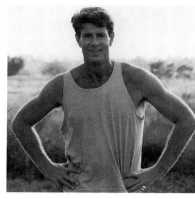

learned that if he didn't take responsibility for his own health and fitness, nobody else would. In the minors he had played for the hard-driving Cal Ripken, Sr., father of future Hall of Famer and Orioles ironman Cal Ripken, Jr. "Everybody ran hard who played for Cal because he made you," Palmer says. "Then, when you got to the big leagues, you were on your own. They thought that since you were in the big leagues, you ought to be able to make conscious decisions that were going to be the right ones. Well, a guy would stay out late drinking or have a headache or didn't feel like running or was a little overweight, and he wouldn't run. And then it would reflect in his performance."

Postgame spreads in major-league locker rooms back then usually featured meat and potatoes, and there were always plenty of candy bars on hand for a quick energy boost. Today, you'll find healthier foods—fruits and vegetables—mixed in with the candy bars, but Palmer says many athletes still have the naive notion that nutrition doesn't matter.

"There's a certain imperviousness to health when you're young and vibrant and full of life," says Palmer, a three-time Cy Young Award winner who chalked up 268 victories en route to being the only pitcher ever to win World Series games in three decades. "You look around and how many guys shortened their careers because they didn't take care of themselves? An unbelievably great amount of them."

Eating for Life

Palmer took great care of himself throughout his playing days but pinpoints a West Coast visit to Hollywood stuntman Ted Grossman's home in 1978 as a real turning point in terms of nutrition. When he checked the food supply there, Palmer recalls, all he saw were fruits, vegetables, nuts and rice. "And I'm going, 'What am I going to eat? This is all healthy stuff.'"

Palmer had eliminated many of the really high-fat items from his diet following his Puerto Rico trip in 1968 but credits his friendship with Grossman with truly opening his eyes to the full

---

Power Eating

Here is a typical day's menu for Jim Palmer.

Breakfast: Mixes several cereals, such as wheat bran, Grape-Nuts, Shredded Wheat and Kashi, topped with a banana. Fresh-baked bread, toasted and plain, and juice.

Lunch: "If I play golf, I usually have fruit and a power bar. Maybe soup or salad. Very rarely will I eat anything but that."

Dinner: "I try to eat early, which is sometimes impossible. If I'm doing a game, I eat light afterward. Maybe a salad or some soup. And I just eat fish or chicken. Maybe beef once a month."

Snacks: Fruit. As an occasional treat, a small portion of Häagen-Dazs vanilla ice cream with a fruit derivative topping, or a Mrs. Field's chocolate chip cookie.

---

benefits of eating for health and nutrition.

He may be a true believer, but he doesn't consider himself to be a fanatic. "Life's too short not to have a Mrs. Field's cookie or some Häagen-Dazs ice cream or whatever," says Palmer, who still lives in Baltimore most of the year with his wife, Joni. "Moderation—that is the key. There are people who are overly zealous about everything, whether it's religion or diet or just work, work, work. It's nice to have a happy, pleasant mix where you can eat health-consciously, but you don't have to overdo it.

Conscious decisions. That's what it all comes down to for Jim Palmer. And all of those little daily decisions add up to one big one: to lead a longer and healthier life.

"I want to live as long as I possibly can. I don't want to know what's after life. That's going to happen soon enough. It's inevitable that that's going to happen. So you make conscious lifestyle decisions."

Kareem Abdul-Jabbar, Hall of Fame Basketball Player

Scoring Points by Eating Right

To see him play for most of his 20 seasons, Kareem Abdul-Jabbar's millions of fans would never guess the basketball legend could ever have to worry about his weight.

"I think most people saw just the opposite—a tall, skinny guy who looked like he could use a good meal," Abdul-Jabbar says. And while that was true for most of his career, in his final basketball season before retirement in 1989 at the age of 42, the former center for the Los Angeles Lakers found himself trying to shed a nagging eight pounds that refused to leave his 7-foot-2 frame.

"A lot of that was just needing to get back into shape for the season after laying off for a few months. But I won't deny that the extra pounds had to get on there some way, and how much I ate was playing a role," he says.

When he was playing basketball, the solution was to double up his training and burn off the extra pounds. But now, as an entrepreneur—the Hall of Famer heads his own company, Kareem Enterprises, in Los Angeles—Abdul-Jabbar says he shares the same fitness concerns of many successful businessmen, namely finding the right time and place to get all the right foods.

"Now I'm traveling all over the world on business," he says. "It does take a bite out of my time for exercise and good eating."

A Sea of Smart Choices

During his playing days Abdul-Jabbar burned calories as routinely as he torched

opposing centers. He retired with the all-time NBA record for most points scored—a staggering 38,387, nearly 7,000 more than the immortal Wilt Chamberlain. He also held the all-time career marks for games played and blocked shots and was third on the all-time rebounding list, behind only Chamberlain and Bill Russell.

Once he stopped running the hardwood floors of basketball arenas night after grueling night, though, Abdul-Jabbar realized he had to change his eating habits.

"Initially, it was hard to make the transition from sports to business, at least in terms of my diet," says Abdul-Jabbar. "When I stopped playing, I started to gain all this weight—all of a sudden I noticed this gut growing on this long frame, and I was just appalled. I was still working out, but I wasn't burning the calories the way I had on the court. I realized then that I had to make modifications."

Abdul-Jabbar started by modifying the portions he was eating—"I just didn't need all that fuel anymore"—and then he focused on sticking to a diet that emphasized lean meats, grains and plenty of fruits and vegetables. "Once you learn what to eat, having a healthy diet—even when you're on the road—is not that tough. Although I'm on the road for many months of the year, I still eat a balanced diet," he says.

A large part of that diet is fresh seafood. "Wherever I am, I try to seek out the local

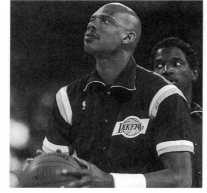

seafood, whatever it is, be it soft-shell crab or salmon. Especially salmon. I love it. I'll even have it for breakfast from time to time," he says.

Enter the Dragon

Abdul-Jabbar isn't content to let 20 years of NBA muscle degenerate into postgame flab. Like most professional athletes, Abdul-Jabbar knows the secret to being fit—and having fewer restrictions on his diet—is to build and keep calorie-burning muscle. "I didn't always feel this way. When I was playing, for a long time it was considered taboo to build up any muscle—players thought it would make them slow," he recalls.

Indeed, Abdul-Jabbar was first pushed to do weight training by a nonbasketball superstar—karate legend Bruce Lee, whom Abdul-Jabbar met during his college days. "He was always pushing me to build muscle, but I resisted him. Eventually, I tried it and noticed a tremendous difference in my game and in my general fitness. If you look at professional athletes today, you know that most of them see the value of it, too. And it helps you off the field as well," he says.

Staying Flexible

Today, Abdul-Jabbar's workout consists of a six-day-a-week cross-training schedule. "It varies day to day—depending on my schedule and how I feel, but I try to do some lifting and some running." Finally, Abdul-Jabbar rounds out his workouts with a yoga routine. "I've been doing stretches since my days with Coach John Wooden when I was at UCLA. Absolutely, that's what allowed me to stay in the game longer than anyone. But even if you've never played professional sports, stretching is a vital part of your total fitness. The more flexible I am, the more I can use my body to do whatever I want."

And it's not like Abdul-Jabbar has retired to a life of leisure. He can still play a little ball. Just ask the Harlem Globetrotters. In September 1995, Abdul-Jabbar led a team of former pro players against the legendary clown princes of basketball. Showing his old

---

Power Eating

"I've always paid special attention to eating because I have first-hand knowledge of how important it is," explains Kareem Abdul-Jabbar. Here's a typical day's menu for the former NBA champion.

Breakfast: Bowl of fresh fruit, two eggs, turkey bacon or sausage, hash browns and apple juice

Lunch: Piece of fruit, turkey sandwich and cranberry juice

Dinner: Shrimp curry, serving of rice, serving of fresh vegetables and cranberry juice

Snacks: Fresh fruit; Ice cream (occasionally)

---

touch, he poured in 34 points on 15-of-16 shooting to lead the Kareem Abdul-Jabbar All-Stars to a 91-85 victory—ending the Trotters's amazing 8,829-game winning streak that dated back to 1971.

The six-time NBA champion realizes that by staying in shape, he can continue to burn calories, even from the foods he knows he shouldn't eat.

Even legendary sports figures have foods they know they should avoid. As a Muslim, Abdul-Jabbar has two important dietary restrictions—no pork and no alcohol. And while that means he never has to worry about getting a beer gut, Abdul-Jabbar does have his weaknesses.

"I love ice cream, oh yes," he confides. "I'll seek it out wherever I am. Overseas, when I was in Italy, I loved the kind they call gelati—I can get into that pretty good if I'm not careful. It's my one guilty pleasure. But you know, after a long day of work you have to give yourself something to shoot for."

As the man who took—and made—more shots than anyone else in NBA history, Abdul-Jabbar ought to know.

Robert Duncan McNeill, Actor

A Trekker's Nutritional Voyage

Robert Duncan McNeill was working as an actor in the center of the universe (New York City) when an alien corner of the galaxy beckoned (take your pick: Los Angeles or the TV series *Star Trek: Voyager*).

The only problem: He needed a body that was a little more, well, celestial.

"When I got the *Star Trek* role, I was in New York doing a play off-Broadway. When producer Rick Berman called to say I had the job, he also called to say, 'We want you to lose some weight. We want you to be the leading man of our show and the lady-killer kind of character, and we need someone who's going to be really trim and in shape.'"

At the time, the six-foot-tall actor weighed more than 200 pounds. During his dozen or so years in the acting profession, McNeill had explored a broad range of roles. He studied for two years at Julliard, and at the same time portrayed Charlie Brent on the popular ABC soap opera *All My Children*. Then came a progression of jobs, which included Stephen Sondheim's *Into the Woods*, John Guarre's *Six Degrees of Separation*, a guest appearance on *Star Trek: The Next Generation*, ABC's *Going to Extremes* and *Homefront* and the CBS comedy *Second Chances*.

And during McNeill's professional voyage he made a discovery: Sometimes the very nature of the job ensures that a guy will keep his lady-killer proportions. And sometimes it doesn't.

"When I was younger, I really didn't have to worry about my health and weight as much," McNeill says. "I also did a lot of musical comedy in New

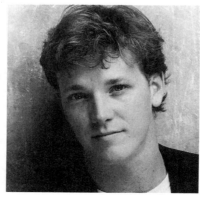

York, so I was dancing and staying in shape. In the past few years I have been doing a lot more television. Combine that with getting older and turning 30, and I started to put on some weight. I didn't have an exercise routine. Because I have two young kids, I tended to be up in the middle of the night a lot. I was eating yogurt and cookies all night, and those middle-of-the-night snacks were just killing me."

To nail down the role of Starfleet pilot Lieutenant Tom Paris, McNeill enlisted the aid of a Los Angeles trainer, Lisa Sanchez. They overhauled what and how McNeill was eating and started him on a six-day-a-week workout routine.

Cleaning Up His Act

McNeill speaks passionately now of "clean" carbohydrates and proteins, meaning sources that are low in fats, oils and simple sugars. Unlike many guys, he was already eating ample amounts of beans, grains and vegetables because his wife and two children are vegetarians. Now he avoids fatty and sugary baked goods and gets extra protein from chicken and fish.

He reduced his salt and caffeine consumption. "I found that a lot of the spices and sauces that I had used had a lot of sodium in them—that I was retaining water," McNeill explains. "I used to drink a lot of coffee—sometimes a whole pot of coffee by noon. That was great for waking up and for getting quick energy, but it also made me crave junk food later. My energy and my blood sugar levles were like a roller coaster—always up and down. Now I just try to have two cups max in the morning, which keeps my moods and my energy level a little more consistent."

He also cut back on one of his great loves: beer. "You don't drive in New York City. So when I was doing theater, after the shows I would go out and have some beer," McNeill says. "I wasn't a big boozer, but three or four nights a week I'd go out and have two or three drinks. Before you know it, that's a lot of calories. So I cut out the casual social drinking. I save it for special occasions—some sort of celebration."

He also tries to drink a lot of water throughout the day. "I find it hard to drink water all day, even though I know it's really good for me," McNeill says. "If I take one of those big liter bottles of water and dump a little Crystal Light in there, I tend to drink it more. There are a few calories in it, but very few."

And there are no more late-night snacks. "My trainer and I have agreed that I will not have anything to eat during the three hours before I go to sleep," McNeill says. "If I know that I'll be in bed at ten o'clock, then seven o'clock is it—nothing after that."

Three or four days a week McNeill lifts weights (a machine circuit plus dumbbells), followed by aerobic exercise. On other workout days he sticks to aerobic exercise—on a stair-climber or a stationary bike. He found that running was best for keeping his waistline under control, but leg troubles have kept him off the track.

A Task for Communicators

Starfleet personnel, of course, have no problem getting exactly the food they want. Make a request and—zoop—dinner materializes instantly on a replicator.

But if you're just an actor putting in 15- to 18-hour workdays, the most you can hope

> ## Power Eating
>
> The following is a typical day's menu for Robert Duncan McNeill.
>
> **Breakfast:** Egg-white omelet or scrambled egg whites, boiled or baked potato, sometimes oatmeal; limited dairy products, and no honey or sugar
>
> **Midmorning Snack:** Apple or celery
>
> **Lunch:** Chicken breast or tuna, pasta or rice on the side
>
> **Midafternoon Snack:** Apple or dried fruit ("I try to snack and keep my cravings down so that I don't go crazy.")
>
> **Dinner:** Salad with a squeeze of lemon (but no dressing), vegetables, chicken or fish
>
> **Late Snack:** No way

for is a cooperative restaurant where you can dine. You do have to assert yourself when dining out, however.

"At a lot of restaurants, I've found that if you tell them how you want something prepared—giving very specific instructions—they'll do it for you," McNeill says. "At first I was very uncomfortable making these requests. People usually hesitate, because it says on the menu that the item comes with a cream sauce: 'Well, there's nothing for me to eat here.' But if you just say, 'Look, pasta. Plain—nothing,' they'll bring you a bowl of nice clean pasta and you can sprinkle a little Parmesan cheese on it.

"Because we have kids who are vegetarians, we often have to ask restaurants to do special things. So between having kids and what I needed to do for my work—you know, to fit into the space suit—I've learned that restaurants will try to accommodate you. It's not a problem."

Jacques Pépin, World-Class Chef

Enjoying His Salad Days

Jacques Pépin does a lot of talking about food. The renowned cooking expert roams the United States for at least 30 weeks out of the year teaching and making appearances. He banters with David Letterman now and then on the *Late Show*, shares secrets with PBS viewers during his *Today's Gourmet* series and speaks to readers from the pages of *Food & Wine* magazine and more than a dozen books, including *Jacques Pépin's Simple and Healthy Cooking.*

So when he's between classes, the TV shows are in the can, all the recipes are written and he's home in Connecticut, what does he do? He talks to himself—about food.

"I would say that it is very important to listen to your body, to what it tells you as you get older," says Pépin, who recently turned 60. "I'm not a macrobiotic guru trying to tell people to get into some type of inner experience. It's really not that complicated."

A Lifelong Love Affair with Food

Pépin grew up in the kitchen. His mother was the chef in the family restaurant near Lyon, France, and as a child, young Jacques was her helper. At age 13, Pépin began his formal apprenticeship as a chef at the Grand Hotel de L'Europe in his hometown.

Eventually, he made his way to the bright lights of Paris, where he continued his training at two of the city's finest restaurants. In the mid-1950s, Pépin served as personal chef to three French heads of state, including the legendary Charles de Gaulle.

In 1959, Pépin decided to seek his fame and fortune

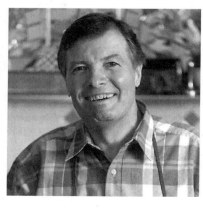

across the Atlantic Ocean. Starting in the kitchen of New York's historic Le Pavillon, he moved on to the Howard Johnson Company, where he served as director of research and new development for ten years. While establishing his reputation as one of the world's most creative and colorful chefs, Pépin earned his master's degree in eighteenth century French literature from Columbia University in New York City.

Changing with the Times

Pépin's philosophy on cooking is still very much rooted in his mother's childhood kitchen.

"I try to eat not much differently than when I was much younger," Pépin says. "When I was a kid living in France, we didn't really eat meat more than once or twice a week. Not because it was a fad or for health purposes—we didn't know anything about that—but probably more because of economic conditions. I was never the type of person who ate a lot of meat every day because I just didn't feel like it."

Over the years, though, Pépin has gradually moved away from using ingredients high in saturated fat and cholesterol, such as butter. He has also cut back considerably on the use of meats and desserts. Part of it has been the growing awareness about what constitutes healthy eating. And part of it has been Pépin's personal journey.

"There has been a great deal of change in the last 20 years or so in the eating habits of people," Pépin notes. "And I feel that I have been part of it, as I have been here doing recipes for many, many years. I would also say that I am 20 years older, and you kind of follow your body, you know?

"I am sure that I am eating things now that I would not have been that crazy about 20 or 30 years ago. It's just that I'm older and I don't feel like eating the same way. I'm eating more soup, more vegetables, things like this, because that's what I feel like eating."

A Matter of Taste

Don't for a moment, however, think that Pépin would sacrifice taste on the altar of low-fat living. He is, first and foremost, a chef. Pépin has not eliminated any ingredients—including butter, beef or sugar—from his kitchen. He has merely scaled them back and found innovative ways to trim the fat while maintaining the flavor.

Pépin believes that chefs should never say never. Take cream sauces, for example. "I haven't seen cream sauce in a restaurant in at least two or three years," Pépin says. "But very often, I have made it on my show to purposely show that it can be done with much fewer calories."

So Pépin will take scrod and mix together a sauce with white wine, horseradish, black olives, and—gasp!—some sour cream.

"Now, it comes out to about one tablespoon of sour cream per person, and that's 20 calories. So it's really nothing much at all, much less than if you had grilled it with olive oil. But the point is that people look at that dish, with the white sauce oozing out of it, and say, 'That's it. I'm dead.' They won't touch it, you know?"

When it comes to eating, Pépin suffers from the same temptations as the rest of us. "I am the type of person who can probably do without a meal, but if it's in front of my nose, I am going to eat it. Which is not necessarily good," he confesses.

The key to healthy eating, Pépin says, is smart shopping.

"I love to go to the market. Unless I have to write a recipe and I go specifically for one thing that I need, I like to see what's good, what's interesting there. I'm talking mostly about vegetables and fruits. I start buying this way, listening to what I feel like eating these days. It's a natural way of doing it. It works for me."

Power Eating

Here is a typical day's menu for Jacques Pépin:

Breakfast: Coffee and fruit juice

Lunch: Bread, cheese and wine

Snack: None, except for the occasional taste while he's cooking

Dinner: Hen, vegetable and noodle soup made from the hen's stock, bread and salad

Dessert: A peach

Pépin is a big fan of salads, and they're tossed together in a similarly intuitive fashion. And the simple fact that fresh salad makings are always easily at hand in his refrigerator makes it more likely that he will make wise eating decisions.

"We had a big salad last night," he says. "I think it was romaine. I opened the refrigerator and I had a piece of cucumber, half a lettuce and half a tomato or whatever, and we used that."

As a rule, Pépin doesn't eat between meals. "That would be very rare. Unless I'm cooking," he says. "But usually, if I have lunch, I do not have anything before dinner. It's not part of the way I live, so I don't try to get bad habits if I don't have them."

And he doesn't care much for dessert either—at least nothing from the oozing-with-chocolate food group. "Last night I had a very nice, ripe peach, so I peeled some and that's what we had for dessert. I mean, most of the time, except for fruit or maybe a piece of cheese, we really don't have dessert."

That's normally something he saves for special occasions. "Very often in our house, that's what makes the difference between an everyday meal and a guest meal," Pépin says. "Because if people come over on the weekend, or we have guests unexpectedly, I may serve the same meal that I was going to serve, but then add a dessert."

You Can Do It! These guys are juggling jobs, families and other important factors—just like you. Although they have different stories to tell, they share at least one thing in common: a commitment to eating right. They're food smart—and you can be, too.

Surviving the Lunch Crowd

John M. Anderson, Columbus, Ohio

Date of birth: January 10, 1937

Height and weight: 5-foot-6, 190 pounds

Profession: Attorney

Favorite junk food: Corned beef

Favorite health food: Turkey

About a year ago my doctor discovered liver enzymes in my blood. He told me there were two possible reasons why the enzymes were there. One could have been a medication I was taking for colitis. The other could have been that I was overweight. Since the medication for my colitis is very important, we decided to try to get rid of the enzymes by controlling my weight.

I changed my eating habits and started exercising. I try to walk four miles a day, four or five days a week. The exercise tends to give you a false sense of security. You think you can take this weight off and keep it off and that leaves you to eat pretty much as you please. And of course that's not true. It would be nice, though. It made me think that now that I'm walking, that's 400 calories free that I can eat. Instead of reducing my weight, I just increased my intake.

But then I started eliminating butter and other fat from my diet. Butter is in everything when you stop and think about it. Most of the time if you eat a piece of bread, you can eat the bread without the butter and it will taste almost as good if it's good bread.

Lunch is the Key

My big problem is that I'm a lawyer and so I go out to lunch a lot. That's my business. I can't really choose a restaurant that I know has healthier food, because the places that are available for eating lunch are sometimes fixed. You have to go where the client goes. I'm not my own master. And most restaurants when you get right down to it serve you what they can make the most profit on. And the things they can make the most profit on are not necessarily healthy foods.

If you can control what you eat for lunch, then you have a better chance of losing weight. I am not totally successful at that, but I do reasonably well. I try to order more healthy foods. One of the things I like more than anything in the world is delicatessen food. But of course they are just about the worst things you can possibly eat. You know—corned beef, pastrami and so forth. So I've been watching that. Sometimes I reward myself, but I try not to be too greedy about it.

I've been able to lose weight. Not as much as I would like, but I've been able to lose 15 pounds. That's my problem. I'm at a plateau and I think it's because I began relying more on the exercise and less on the diet. I haven't made enough changes in my diet. I would like to lose 15 more pounds.

I think if I can find a way to control even more of what I eat for lunch and avoid second helpings more often, I would be able to start losing weight again. I've tried to avoid second helpings, but my wife, Deb, is a good cook. She cooks healthy food, but we always have generous portions. She and I laugh about that.

Mastering Energy

Ed Marshall,
Kirkland, Washington

Date of birth: February 19, 1947

Height and weight: 5-foot-9, 150 pounds

Profession: Mechanical engineer for Seattle City Light. Also operates Ed Marshall Financial Navigator, a financial mentoring service.

Favorite junk food: "I can't think of anything. The last time I had a Twinkie was 20 years ago."

Favorite health food: Fish and rice

I weigh exactly the same today that I weighed when I graduated from high school. It never changes, and the reason is that there's a consistency in my approach: Energy in and energy out.

I don't believe diets work—I believe in lifestyle. When you indulge in a bad habit, do so in moderation. Let the bulk of what you consume be food that is beneficial to you—which, by the way, is a parallel to my financial philosophy. Things that increase your personal worth should be your lifestyle.

When I'm hungry, I eat. It sounds simplistic, but it's not. On a typical day I'll eat six, seven or eight pieces of fruit simply because I'm feeding myself when I'm hungry. I eat two or three main meals a day, and I try to have them in a standardized time frame. It doesn't always happen that way, but when it doesn't, I can substitute a banana or a peach.

I eat breakfast at five or six in the morning, while I'm working as a financial navigator, my mentoring service. I typically have coffee, a vitamin C, a high-grain, low-sugar cereal and maybe a piece of fruit. Dairy is a minuscule portion of my diet because I'm dairy intolerant.

When I arrive at my 9-to-6 job, I guess you might call that my extended breakfast. I'll grab as many as three pieces of fruit, depending on how active I am that morning—an apple, an orange, grapes.

Eating and Relaxation

For lunch I take a full hour every single day. It's not just eating time—lunch is a relaxed state of mind as well as a relaxed state of body.

I eat fish and rice for lunch. There's a large, diverse Asian community here in Seattle, so I can do fish and rice in many ways: Vietnamese, Chinese, Japanese. As a result, I have extremely good cholesterol levels—a high HDL and a low LDL.

During the afternoon it's more fruit—grapes, figs, prunes, peaches, oranges, apples. Fortunately, I live in an agricultural state. The quantities of produce that are available are just overwhelming. I also work about four blocks from the Pike Place Market, a traditional open-air market that carries anything and everything I want.

When I arrive home in the evening I do some chill-down mental activities such as personal planning or just lying down. Then, three or four times a week, I stick on some running shoes and do about a 10-K. As you can see, I'm consuming an enormous amount of bulk, which is a natural response to all of the calories that I burn.

I eat supper after 8:00 P.M., and on the nights that I run, it will be small, something as simple as soup, a sandwich and a salad. Maybe once a week I'll have a big sit-down dinner, pot roast or something, typically game that I have harvested myself. Game meat is low-fat, and the wok cooking I like to do is low-fat, so when you combine the two, you reliably get a low-fat meal. I eat for taste. I eat until I'm *not hungry*. I don't eat until I'm full. Just as with your financial endeavors, you have to have a plan—to know where you're headed.

Healthy for the Long Haul

Dave Dobransky, New Albany, Indiana

Date of birth: May 3, 1950

Height and weight: 5-foot-8, 190 pounds

Profession: Over-the-road truck driver

Favorite junk food: Ice cream

Favorite health food: Low-fat yogurt

My wife, Julie, and I are over-the-road truck drivers. We move high-value products, such as art work, computers, things for the military and medical fields. It can be anything from a Matisse to part of a satellite.

We've been working this way for 11 years now, and this is the fourth truck we've owned, a 1995 Peterbilt. We're forunate—it's considered a luxury truck, with a shower and toilet, refrigerator, microwave, TV, VCR, a sleeper. It's more or less a small efficiency apartment.

I started putting on weight, even though we work very hard. My age might have had something to do with it, but I think the main problem was that I was eating the same things I always had but I wasn't exercising like I used to.

We tried diets—this much intake of calories, this for lunch. I've done it countless times over the years and it *never* worked. Oh, one time I dropped from 220 pounds down to 165 with a combination of strenuous exercises and dieting.

But after a while I crept back up to 200 pounds and the battle began again.

There were two big influences that finally led me to realize the significance of a proper diet—my wife and *Prevention* magazine. After reading *Prevention* and seeing how important controlling your fat intake is— not only for your weight but for your general health as far as cancer risks, heart attacks and cholesterol—we realized this was something we had to do.

A Daily Plan

When I get up, say at 6:00 or 7:00 A.M., I'll always have some type of fresh fruit. Grapefruit is really our favorite, or a cantaloupe. We'll also have either a bagel or an English muffin. Julie bakes nonfat apple-cinnamon muffins and blueberry muffins. Or we'll have cereal with fresh fruit such as strawberries or bananas.

Around 10 or 10:30 we'll have a snack, anything from a banana to a pear, to low-fat cookies or chips.

For lunch we have a variety of things. It may be soup, it may be sandwiches with nonfat cheeses and low-fat lunchmeat— bologna, turkey, ham—low-fat Ramen noodle soups from Campbell's or entrées from Lean Cuisine.

We eat dinner anywhere from 5:00 to 8:00 P.M. We target restaurants such as Ponderosa, Sizzler, Shoney's, Denny's, places that offer you low-fat options such as fish or grilled chicken or salad bars. We usually don't eat dessert at the restaurant because the options there are still back in the Ice Age. We rely on our muffins or Entenmann's fat-free, cholesterol-free, fruit-flavored Danish twists, available in lemon or raspberry flavors. We always try to stock something like that so if a sweet temptation hits, we use that.

So that's all I eat for the day until, say, it's my turn to go to bed about 9:00 P.M., and then I get up at 2:00 or 3:00 in the morning and start to drive. Then I'll have another piece of fruit.

I honestly believe that a person who makes an effort can control a lot of what happens to his health over the years. I have a plan. I would like to retire when I'm a young man and golf and fish and travel. But man, if you don't have your health, none of this is worth it.

Battling High Cholesterol

Paul Folkman, Mansfield, Massachusetts

Date of birth: November 2, 1954

Height and weight: 5-foot-11, 175 pounds

Profession: Real estate developer, builder

Favorite junk food: Goldfish crackers

Favorite health food: Pears

About four years ago we had some heart-related deaths in the family. A lightbulb went on, and I had my cholesterol checked. It was running up into the 330s. It was extremely elevated.

I didn't want to use cholesterol-lowering medications because their long-term impacts just weren't known. So my doctor and I looked at lowering my cholesterol levels by changing my diet.

My wife, Jane, and I have changed our diet substantially from a meat-and-potatoes orientation to a lot less emphasis on that. But we did it slowly. We gradually cut back from eating red meat three times a week to just once a week. Then we started changing portion sizes. Before, I would sit down and eat a ten-ounce sirloin strip steak. Later, one day we looked at each other and started laughing because we were using a strip and a half for me, Jane and the three kids, Erin, Alicia and David. We were just slicing it up, stir-frying it and having it with pasta.

The cholesterol numbers went down. Then another lightbulb went on in my brain and I started an exercise regimen. I did that slowly, too. I started out with the stationary bike and a stair-climber and worked my way up to a treadmill and cross-country ski machine.

Then I worked my way up to outside biking and running. When I weighed 210 pounds, I could hardly stay on the stair-climber. Now, I can run five or six miles. That may not sound like a lot to some people, but for someone who 3½ years ago couldn't stay on the stair-climber for ten minutes, that's a big deal.

I think what's hard for people when they first start is that they have all these images in magazines of the people at the end point who can climb mountains and do all these things. It's a longer process.

A Reformed Junk-Food Junkie

Five years ago I was the classic fast-food person. I would go through Wendy's or the McDonald's drive-throughs on my busy days. Other days, I just went out to lunch. For the first year of this diet, I substituted the workout time for the lunch time. At that time, I was going to work out at five minutes to noon, so instead of eating lunch, I would have a snack in the late morning. Then I would work out. Once I broke the habit of going to lunch and thinking of fast food, I had a little more willpower and I was able to move my gym time to later in the afternoon so it was more convenient. It works for me.

It's really weird because even when we go out to eat now, I eat differently. Usually if you are going out to dinner, you reward yourself. I used to never order chicken or fish. I would have the prime rib. I'm different now, but it has taken some time. Five, six years ago I would go out and have fish and chips. If I try to eat that today, I get sick. Sometimes I eat something and I don't know it has a high-fat content and I get a reaction to it. Now my body's much more sensitive to that kind of junk.

The doctor would like to have my cholesterol count in the low 200s. I'm still around the 260s. He and I are in agreement not to go into the heavy drugs, so we're going to experiment with a little more fiber.

Male Makeovers

Eating right can be tough in today's fast-paced world. There are a dizzying array of choices, and it's not always easy to make the correct one. Our experts give their advice on how to be food smart.

On the Fast Track, Running Out of Fuel

The Scenario

Albert figures he's a realist: At age 52, a guy's pretty well destined to have a paunch, a flagging sex drive and low energy.

He gets three square meals on most days. Breakfast is usually eggs, sausage, an English muffin and coffee. Lunch is often meat loaf or a burger in the company cafeteria. For dinner fried chicken and mashed potatoes is a favorite.

His wife has gotten used to his late hours at work and doesn't serve dinner until 9:00 P.M. She tried to talk nutrition with Albert a couple of times, but a life of fish and asparagus isn't his idea of living at all.

He considers himself pretty healthy, unless you want to count recurring constipation and spells of midafternoon drowsiness.

The Solution

Albert is living the stressed-out corporate lifestyle, and consequently his diet suffers. Most of all, Albert needs to learn to add some color to his plate—particularly in the form of fruits and vegetables.

Let's look at Albert's breakfast. Judging from his eating pattern, it's a good bet that he fries his eggs in oil, eats the sausage he's served, puts margarine or butter on his English muffin and possibly even adds creamer to his coffee. This fat overload in the morning doesn't provide the proper energy for his body. He would be better off working in some fresh fruit and yogurt or milk in the morning, combined with lower-fat protein alternatives, or whole-wheat toast or whole-grain cereal.

A glance at his lunch and dinner tells you Albert is a meat-and-potatoes, fast-food kind of guy. With this eating approach, Albert is ensuring himself a high-fat intake and a lack of vitamins A and C, which mainly come from fruits and vegetables.

The late meals are working against him, too. The later a person eats in the evening, the more fat he stores from that meal. And with each pound of fat he gains, he adds an estimated 200 miles of blood vessels to his circulatory system, which taxes the heart.

Given Albert's neglect of his nutrition, it's a fair assumption that he's ignoring his intake of water, which is considered to be one of the six essential nutrients. Being dehydrated can cause sluggishness and fatigue, which could contribute to his lack of energy. Drinking plenty of water would also help him maintain an ideal body weight. He should try to drink at least six to eight eight-ounce glasses of water a day.

Just as we have to fuel our cars properly, so must we fuel our bodies from the inside out for increased nutritional benefits and overall wellness.

—Tammi R. Wolosuk, R.D., San Diego

Gaining Weight and Losing Time

The Scenario

In Wayne's house it seems as if food is always at the center of one crisis or another. For one thing, both he and his wife work Monday through Friday, which means preparing dinner is a nightly hassle. Wayne's solution: He finds a frozen dinner he likes, a Chinese stir-fry, and he pulls one of those out of the freezer sometimes for variety. He wouldn't mind a salad or a vegetable, too, but that's more work than he has time for.

Now in his midthirties, Wayne has noticed that his waistline has expanded a couple of inches in the last few years. Also, his doctor is starting to grumble about high blood pressure, but Wayne figures he'll worry about that when he turns 40.

The Solution

There's no reason Wayne should wait until he's in his forties to work on preventing high blood pressure. Here are some simple steps he can begin with now.

- Lose weight. Even as little as ten pounds can have a favorable impact on his blood pressure.
- Exercise. For starters, if he drives to work, he could park his car farther away and walk several blocks to the office. If he takes a bus or train, he could get off a stop early or a stop late and walk. Once he starts getting his body in gear,

increasing his activity level is not as difficult. It's always the beginning of an exercise program that people dread. (Always check with your doctor before starting any exercise program.)

- Limit sodium intake. The recommendation is that everyone should keep sodium intake below 2,400 milligrams per day.

With prepared dinners like the frozen stir-fry that Wayne likes, it's very important to check the sodium on the nutrition label. A rule of thumb: Allow about 600 milligrams per meal. Three meals a day, then, would amount to 1,800 milligrams, leaving a margin of 600 milligrams for snacks and such.

Say he decides to have his Chinese stir-fry and it fits in with his sodium requirements. To make it a little bit more nutritious, he could start dropping by the supermarket salad bars on the way home so he can have his fresh vegetables.

An alternative: Stock up on frozen vegetables—they're better than canned vegetables, which commonly have added sodium. Frozen foods are very simple: You open the bag and put them in boiling water or microwave them. In the time it takes him to prepare his stir-fry, he can have his vegetables ready, too. Add a slice of whole-wheat bread to get some fiber and a glass of skim milk to make it more nutritious. For dessert: fresh fruit. This doesn't mean he can't have sugary snacks also, but he should get some fruit in first.

What I recommend is a little organization to help their hectic lives. On the weekend, they could write up a shopping list for what they will need during the week. Most of us have a select amount of meals that we eat over and over again, so this is not really a lot of prep work. During the week, they'll have all the ingredients they need and will avoid extra trips to the grocery store. Also, when they cook on the weekends, they can make double the amount they want to eat and freeze the rest for use during the week.

—Agnes Kolor, R.D., Pearl River, New York

Living in the Fast-Food Lane

The Scenario

John, single and in his midtwenties, is always on the go. And so is his food. Because he's either racing off to or coming home exhausted from touch football, pickup basketball and weight lifting, John often eats out, mostly at fast-food restaurants. When he eats in, he survives primarily on box-to-mouth food—chips and salsa, doughnuts, sometimes spaghetti. And barely a meal goes by without meat. His motto: Lots of protein, lots of muscles. His idea of eating vegetables begins—and ends—with the tomato and iceberg lettuce they put on his cheeseburger.

The Solution

John is fortunate because an active man in his twenties can consume the most calories ever in his life span without gaining extra body fat. He probably knows he might play touch football for a little bit longer, but it's not going to be for the rest of his life. So, developing habits for foods that lack essential nutrients and are high in fat might place him at a high risk for diseases such as diabetes and heart disease.

Since foods high in complex carbohydrates are the primary source of muscle fuel, John's menu choices should include lots of breads, bagels, cereals, pastas, rice, beans, fruits and vegetables. Carbohydrate calories should be 60 percent of his total calories for the day. Protein is the nutrient responsible for building and repairing cell tissue, but extra protein does not build muscle bulk. Exercise does. Unless John is planning to compete at an Olympic event or enter a bodybuilding contest, his protein intake should be 15 percent of his total calories.

Fast foods can be healthy. John should choose sandwiches prepared with lean meats, request no mayonnaise and double the lettuce and tomato. A side salad with low-fat dressing or handfuls of raw vegetables to munch with his sandwich and a carton of low-fat milk would balance the meal. A stop at the grocery store for a bunch of bananas and a sack of apples would supply the vitamins he is presently missing.

There are a lot of foods out of a box that could meet his needs, but sometimes they have a lot of fat. Foods in the box-to-mouth category with better quality would be cereals, fruit juices, bagels with reduced-fat cheese, pretzels, granola bars, puddings, popcorn and reduced-fat tortilla chips with salsa.

Canned foods with no salt added, such as green beans, carrots and beets, are absolutely wonderful for helping with vegetables. Just open the can and mix them together, marinate them or just put a little bit of fat-free Italian dressing on them. The same thing can be done with frozen vegetables. John and other young people who are busy just don't have time to chop and peel fresh vegetables.

Other fast-food options for mealtimes would be the wide variety of nutritious frozen meals available to pop in the microwave. Since many of these meals contain small portions, consider purchasing the larger portions or supplementing the meals with more vegetables and a couple of rolls. Most meals will need additional fruit and also some milk to drink.

It is very important for John to plan in regular mealtimes that contain the energy foods he needs to fuel his muscles for his active lifestyle.

—Diane Wilke, R.D., a nutrition consultant in Columbus, Ohio

Watching His Health Go Up in Smoke

The Scenario

Jason needs every ounce of energy to stay on top of his middle-management job. Married and in his forties, he fears one day being handed one of those corporate-downsizing pink slips. But he does need to down-size himself. He has gained 20 pounds since he began downing chocolate doughnuts, candy bars, M & M'S and soda in an effort to propel himself through the day. And he's still smoking cigarettes, afraid that quitting would add even more pounds around his spare tire.

The Solution

Waving good-bye to smoking doesn't have to mean hello to a spare tire. Jason needs to be informed that it is likely he can quit without gaining weight. But, he may gain weight if he eats more (such as eating five or six slices of pizza rather than three or four) or changes the types of foods he eats (such as indulging in french fries rather than enjoying a baked potato).

A decrease in metabolism may occur upon quitting smoking. If, however, Jason takes a five-minute walking break instead of each five-minute smoking break, he can overcome the potential negative effect of metabolism changes. And he may even cope better with his stressful corporate job.

If his hunger increases after he quits, he'll want to keep his hands busy, find alternative activities to fill spare time and have raw vegetables available for compulsive munching.

He also may want to be more aware of his coffee drinking. Often people have their cigarettes over a cup of coffee. And when they quit, the coffee reminds them of the cigarette. Jason should be prepared for a smoking urge when he has his coffee. Or he could try drinking water instead.

To combat a 20-pound weight gain and further potential weight gain, Jason doesn't have to give up his favorite goodies. He does, however, need to limit the amount and frequency of his "empty calorie" choices. He may benefit from taking cereal bars, raw veggies or fruit to work. These high-carbohydrate foods will give him the energy he needs—as well as balanced nutrition.

Sometimes people who stop smoking get constipated. If that happens, Jason should work some high-fiber foods into his diet. Good fiber-filled food choices include cereals made from whole grains, produce and beans.

But not too fast. Too many changes at once may backfire. So focusing on one change at a time is important for Jason. Smoking cessation alone is a challenge. If he quits smoking today, perhaps two to three months from now he can begin focusing on his office snacking habits and on other major diet or exercise changes.

In the meantime, he and his wife may be able to take minor steps in decreasing fat calories at home without giving up enjoyment. He and his wife can switch from whole milk to 2 percent to 1 percent or skim milk. They can spread jelly on toast instead of fat-laden butter. And they can slightly decrease portion sizes. Following a nutritionally balanced healthy eating plan based on the Food Guide Pyramid is important, too.

Finally, Jason needs to keep moving. Staying active is a key to lifelong weight management.

—Jackie Newgent, R.D., a food, nutrition and wellness consultant in Chicago and contributing author of Cut the Fat

Index

Note: <u>Underscored</u> page references indicate boxed text. **Boldface** references indicate tables.